Strength Ball Training

Lorne Goldenberg
Peter Twist

P9-DFC-277

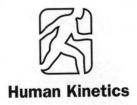

Human Kinetics

Library of Congress Cataloging-in-Publication Data

Goldenberg, Lorne, 1962-
   Strength ball training/Lorne Goldenberg and Peter Twist.
      p. cm.
   Includes bibliographical references and index.
   ISBN 0-7360-3828-0
      1. Weight training. 2. Exercise. 3. Balls (Sporting Goods) I. Twist, Peter, 1963-II.
   Title.
   GV484 .G65 2001
   613.7'1--dc21   2001024448

ISBN: 0-7360-3828-0

Copyright © 2002 by Lorne Goldenberg and Peter Twist

All rights reserved. Except for use in a review, the reproduction or utilization of this work in any form or by any electronic, mechanical, or other means, now known or hereafter invented, including xerography, photocopying, and recording, and in any information storage and retrieval system, is forbidden without the written permission of the publisher.

Acquisitions Editor: Martin Barnard; **Managing Editor:** Wendy McLaughlin; **Assistant Editor:** Dan Brachtesende; **Copyeditor:** Lisa Sheltra; **Proofreader:** Coree Schutter; **Graphic Designer:** Robert Reuther; **Graphic Artists:** Dody Bullerman and Tara Welsch; **Cover Designer:** Keith Blomberg; **Photographer (cover):** Tom Roberts; **Photographer (interior):** Tom Roberts; **Art Manager:** Craig Newsom; **Artist:** Tom Roberts; **Printer:** Versa Press

Human Kinetics books are available at special discounts for bulk purchase. Special editions or book excerpts can also be created to specification. For details, contact the Special Sales Manager at Human Kinetics.

Printed in the United States of America   10 9 8 7 6

Human Kinetics
Web site: www.HumanKinetics.com

United States: Human Kinetics, P.O. Box 5076, Champaign, IL 61825-5076
800-747-4457
e-mail: humank@hkusa.com

Canada: Human Kinetics, 475 Devonshire Road, Unit 100, Windsor, ON N8Y 2L5
800-465-7301 (in Canada only)
e-mail: orders@hkcanada.com

Europe: Human Kinetics, 107 Bradford Road, Stanningley
Leeds LS28 6AT, United Kingdom
+44 (0) 113 255 5665
e-mail: hk@hkeurope.com

Australia: Human Kinetics, 57A Price Avenue, Lower Mitcham, South Australia 5062
08 8277 1555
e-mail: liahka@senet.com.au

New Zealand: Human Kinetics, P.O. Box 105-231, Auckland Central
09-523-3462
e-mail: hkp@ihug.co.nz

Contents

Preface

Swiss and medicine ball strength training have already made valuable contributions to the fields of sport, fitness, and injury rehabilitation. After you read this book, strength training with these balls can become one of the most successful tools for your athletes and clients. It will inject some much-needed variety into traditional weight-training programs, and, when you finally get through this book of more than 60 exercises and see how simple they really are, you will ask yourself, *Why haven't I tried this before?*

The next question you may ask is, *Why would anyone want to get on a ball to perform strength-training exercises?* The answer: An unstable environment is created when a ball is used as the platform for the exercises we describe. To some, this is a negative result. To many, this variable of instability may very well be a key to increased strength levels.

At the time of this writing, the rationale behind this theory has not been proven in a lab, but it does come as a result of our practical experience with hundreds of NHL players as well as elite youth and adult athletes from other sports. We have implemented Swiss and medicine ball training in our development programs for athletes in basketball, soccer, football, rugby, volleyball, powerlifting, baseball, figure skating, skiing, tennis, and lacrosse. In addition to our own experiences, we are also aware of other strength coaches whose athletes have benefited greatly from Swiss and medicine ball training.

There are coaches and trainers who believe the idea of training in an unstable environment is worthless and a dangerous waste of time. Our response? Try it—you'll like it. Strength training with the Swiss and medicine ball is a tool for enhancing your total program. This book is not meant to be the one and only way to train; rather, it's something to use to enhance your own periodized programs and to assist your athletes and clients over strength-training plateaus. We have also used it successfully for injury rehabilitation and re-injury prevention. There is no doubt that training in an unstable environment is much more sport-specific than training in a stable environment; it helps to prepare athletes to meet the demands of their unique circumstances. Sports with unpredictable situations or plays, interaction with teammates, counteraction to opponents, read-and-react situations, or body contact all force the athlete's body into unstable positions.

Training with Swiss and medicine balls helps link your entire body together so that it will work as a functional unit to contribute to sports actions. In this way, it is performance enhancing. But it is also life-specific training. Playing with grandchildren, carrying groceries, helping a friend move furniture, slipping on ice, walking on uneven ground, and countless other regular life occurrences require a body that is capable of linked strength and balance. Without it, you can be injured or completely unable to participate in a simple activity. Most functional restrictions are not a result of aging or disease—they are the result of years of sedentary lifestyle or inadequate fitness training. You can help empower your clients to enjoy a fuller life while remaining injury-free!

This book is not meant to be a scientific explanation justifying the use of Swiss and medicine balls in the weight room. Although there is a short chapter on the muscle mechanics of proprioceptive exercise, the purpose of this book is purely demonstrative. In lectures where we have presented these relatively new techniques, the delegates have always wanted something they could take to the gym to refer to. Well, this is it. We hope that you find it useful!

Acknowledgments

The one person who has had the biggest effect on my career path is Jacques Martin, head coach of the Ottawa Senators. In 1987 he provided me with an opportunity for my first NHL job. Since that time he has not only presented me with additional opportunities, but he has also demonstrated to me the necessary requirements for success in sport and business—perseverance, dedication, understanding, and commitment. Jacques was the jump-start for my professional career and continues to be the successful and respected coach I aspire to be.

When I met Gary Roberts of the Toronto Maple Leafs in 1985, he was a 17-year-old player who did not understand how conditioning could contribute to success on the ice. I was able to convince him that if he worked hard, it would pay dividends in his hockey future. Gary gave me my first opportunity to work with a player headed for the NHL. This opportunity has developed into a great working relationship and lasting friendship that has spanned 16 years. His hard work and perseverance are characteristics that every player should admire. This hard work has led him to be recognized as one as one of the best-conditioned players in the NHL.

The University of Ottawa provided me with an understanding of the human body and an appreciation for the never-ending challenge of education. The National Strength and Conditioning Association has been an avenue to help me with the ability to bridge the gap between science and practice. Since I have attended just about every conference since 1987, the NSCA has played a significant role in developing my coaching abilities. There are other professionals who have shared their systems and philosophies. Charles Poliquin, a fellow Ottawa-born strength coach, who has the ability to turn an underachiever into a champion, has shared many of his concepts and personal thoughts on physical development over the years. Paul Chek made me believe that evaluations were more than skin-caliper and flexibility measurements and also introduced me to my first Swiss ball.

Some of my best friendships have developed as a result of my association in hockey and coaching. Peter Twist is THE source for new and innovative ideas about training for hockey. We have certainly spent many hours discussing the value of optimizing training systems for our sport. Our most valued conversations generally happened at NSCA conferences where the discussion eventually led to where we should go that evening. Peter also happened to be the social convenor for the hockey strength coaches and was always prepared to offer us the best places for a cool one. He is very well rounded in exercise physiology and entertainment! Coaches such as E.J. McGuire, Don Jackson, Mike Keenan, Marc Crawford, and Pierre Page have enriched me with coaching philosophies and support over the years.

R.J. Kamatovic and Sarah Abboud, who were our models for this book, did an excellent job posing and sticking positions. This was very physically demanding on both of them, as attempting to be dynamic yet static was certainly a challenge. I know both of them were quite stiff the next day.

Silvia Reugger from Brooks Canada was very generous in providing Peter, me, and our models, R.J. and Sarah, with some great athletic wear.

This book could not have been completed without the support of my family. Special thanks to my best friend and wife, Julie, who continually puts up with my arriving home late from the gym or office and has to prepare dinner on her own for our two beautiful children, Isaak and Danielle. Without you, I could not have accomplished all of this.

Lorne Goldenberg

I am certainly indebted to the many educators who have positively influenced my own learning, many of whom are affiliated with the National Strength and Conditioning Association—the coaches and exercise specialists who conduct research, pen articles, and share ideas at conferences, all of which help build and improve the field.

Kenner Collegiate Mary Rawlings stimulated my interest in kinesiology; McMaster University's Nick Cipriano turned me on to applying the sport sciences to the coaching process; University of B.C.'s Dr. Ted Rhodes, coauthor of my first book, emphasized physiology and bioenergetics theory; and Dr. Bob Schutz taught me much about academic integrity and meticulous research methodology.

I must mention my coauthor, Lorne Goldenberg, who develops progressive ideas built on attention to research and applies them to the practical sport and exercise setting. Carlos Santana has been innovative and enthusiastic in the design and implementation of exercises. Alex McKechnie is a sport physiotherapist who has embraced functional and active rehab to bridge the gap between injury, rehab, exercise, and game readiness. Current Vancouver Canucks president and general manager Brian Burke, who supports the educational process and contributes to it himself, and David Nonis and Steve Tambellini, who round out the Canucks' management team, have readily shared their player development ideas. Coaches Marc Crawford, Mike Johnston, and Jack McIlhargey have all influenced my coaching philosophy and athlete development style.

Peter Twist

Introduction

To appreciate the power of Swiss and medicine ball training, you must only understand that your body functions together as a unit, with muscles firing sequentially to produce the desired movement; some muscles must contract to help produce movement, some contract to help balance the body; and others contract to stabilize the spine and hold it in a safe, neutral position. Still other muscles kick in each time your body recognizes a shift in position or needs to correct an error, such as when it detects a loss of balance. Your body is a linked system that works together to coordinate athletic actions. Throwing a football relies on the legs, torso, and upper-body muscles, all working together and contracting in the correct sequence. Your body functions as a linked system in everyday life too, such as when you bend over to pick up a baby and lift the baby overhead to produce a smile. This action depends on leg, torso, and upper-body muscles, all prime movers and stabilizers.

However, typical strength training attempts to develop the body with a piecemeal approach, by isolating specific muscle groups. Worse yet, this is often done with the body completely unloaded, sitting stationary on a machine while moving one isolated body part through a controlled range of motion. This type of training has so little relation to real life that it has left participants ill-prepared to meet the demands of both life and sport. Participants often experience more frequent injury and lowered performance from non-functional training.

Over the years, we have improved our strength programs using one-leg dumbbell lifts; medicine ball drills to activate the entire body; and multi-joint, full-body exercises with free weights that incorporate the entire body. However, the most powerful tools have proved to be the Swiss and medicine balls. Strength training with Swiss and medicine balls offer an exciting breakthrough: the opportunity to utilize your body as a unit to execute an exercise.

Most important, you are now training on a round, unstable surface. Your most important feats of strength and balance will be required in unstable, unpredictable environments: slipping on icy stairs, lunging to catch a falling child, withstanding a check while running to catch a lacrosse ball. These real-life situations require contributions from all muscle groups. Each joint and muscle senses its position in space and links to other joints and muscles to react, producing the appropriate action. This linked system is a kinetic chain and safely produces functional movement.

Swiss and medicine ball training builds your body as a unit. It produces improvements that support athletic, dynamic movements such as skiing down a mountain and full-body activities such as digging in a garden. Improve performance and reduce the risk of injury. Improve balance. Build a strong back and strong abdomen. This can all be accomplished with these balls.

Both Swiss and medicine balls are making positive contributions to the fields of sport rehabilitation, athlete conditioning, and general fitness. However, as in all exercise, well-executed technique produces optimal results, while poor technique at best gains nothing and, at worst, often leads to injury. Moving on a ball seems like a simple and playful concept, but activating your body's proprioceptive mechanisms and challenging your low back and deep abdominal stabilizers are important and serious undertakings. An illustrative book demonstrating effective exercises and proper techniques is long overdue. Coaches, trainers, therapists, and self-guided fitness enthusiasts alike can follow the exercise progressions and modifications to customize each exercise for their level of fitness.

The bottom line? You are only as strong as your weakest link. For most people this link is core, or torso, strength. How many people do you know with low back pain? How many athletes have experienced abdominal, hip flexor, and groin strains? Strong legs and strong arms with a weak core are an injury in the making. Swiss and medicine ball training builds from the core out to the periphery, accommodating your upper and lower body while turning your core into your area of strength. A stronger core is both your speed center and strength center. Most movements are initiated and supported with the core muscles—not just your superficial, six-pack muscles, but the more important deep abdominal wall muscles that serve to protect your spine and stabilize movement. The demands and mechanics of swinging a golf club are perfect examples. A golf swing utilizes mostly core muscle strength, a little leg strength, and even less upper-body strength.

Best of all, Swiss and medicine ball exercises are fun to do. As coach, trainer, or athlete you and your participants are more likely to respond positively and stick to a strength ball training program. Take advantage of these powerful tools and get to the core of the matter with Swiss and medicine ball workouts.

Exercise Finder

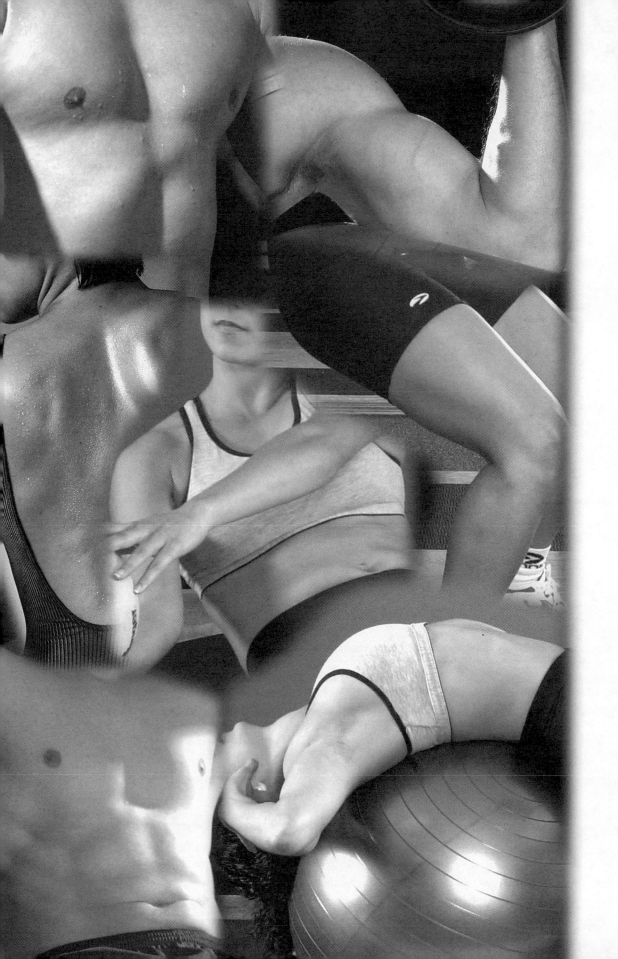

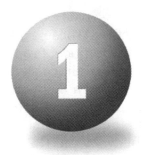

Strength Ball Advantages

The Swiss ball, also known as the stability ball, is currently evolving as a leading-edge exercise modality, but the use of a ball in exercise actually dates back to the second century A.D. "Exercising with a ball can stir the enthusiast or the slacker, it can exercise the lower portions of the body or the upper, some particular part rather than the whole, or it can exercise all the parts of the body equally," explained a Greek philosopher and physician. Most important, he added, "The best athletics of all are those that not only exercise the body but are able to please the spirit" (Posner-Mayer 1995).

Today's Swiss ball was originally developed in the early 1960s as a toy for children. It was adopted by physiotherapists as a means of improving proprioception and balance in their patients (Posner-Mayer 1995). There are a variety of physiological mechanisms that allow Swiss ball training to generate positive results. The physiology is also applicable to strength programs and athlete development, with particular utility for the strength and conditioning professional or the personal trainer. This section provides a brief review of this physiology.

The human body is an amazing machine with many sensory capabilities that allow us to carry out proper motor function. These sensory capabilities can all be described by the term *proprioception*. Proprioception can be thought of as a variety of sensory capabilities that include the sensations of joint movement and joint position (Lephart et al. 1998). It contributes to the motor programming of the neuromuscular control required for precision movements, and it also contributes to muscle reflex, providing dynamic joint stability (McGill 1998).

Excellent proprioceptive capabilities are evident when an athlete has the ability to absorb a hit on the ice or playing field and maintain balance. This is a result of the firing of muscles both at the optimal time and in the correct order. For this to actually take place, there are a number of physiological events that must occur inside the muscle.

There are receptors all over our bodies—in our skin, tendons, and muscles—that react when they sense a change to the tissue. This change is computed by the central nervous system, and, after the brain decides how to react, the proper signals for muscle contraction, and hence movement, are sent to the muscles through the spinal cord and nerves.

There are specific muscles that have many more sensory capabilities than others. The rotator and intertransversarii muscles, for example, are very small segmental muscles in the spine. They cannot produce a high level of force but are very efficient at sensing vertebral position, as they are rich in muscle spindles. Muscle spindles are sensitive to length and rate of stretch and will cause a muscle contraction when their threshold is reached. These two spinal muscles, because of their minimal cross-sectional area, act as position transducers for each lumbar joint, enabling the motor control system to control overall lumbar posture and avoid injury (McGill 1998). This is important in the spine and other articular structures during extreme ranges of movement, as these muscles and neighboring ligaments provide neurological feedback that directly mediates reflex muscular stabilization around the joint (Lephart et al. 1997). For instance, all the segmental muscles must contract to help stabilize the spine during movement. This movement may be the result of performing some conscious act, or as a reaction to a hit on the playing field or a sudden change in the ground underfoot while walking. As you will learn, Swiss and medicine ball training helps the body produce more appropriate unconscious movement, and often means the difference between regaining control and balance and suffering an injury.

Muscle spindles are receptors that mediate the response to plyometric exercise. When stretched at a particular rate and length, they will detect the change, send a signal to the spinal cord, and receive a direct response initiating a reflex contraction in the muscle. This produces a very powerful concentric muscle contraction (Chu 1992). This process is known as the *myotatic stretch reflex*. Here's how it works: The extrafusal (EF) muscle fibers contract or elongate to produce movement. Intrafusal (IF) muscle fibers run parallel to the EF fibers, where they are well positioned to report on the magnitude and rate of muscle lengthening and tension. When the EF fibers quickly elongate, the IF fibers stretch along with them, sending a message to the spinal cord to inhibit the agonist and powerfully contract the stretched muscle. This result is produced quickly because the message travels directly to the spinal cord and back, without taking the longer journey up to the brain.

The golgi tendon organ (GTO) is another type of receptor that is found in the body, more specifically in the musculotendinous junction. The GTO is attached end to end with extrafusal muscle fibers so that it can monitor and respond to tension in a muscle and its tendon. If a GTO reaches its threshold, it will send an inhibitory signal that causes the muscle to relax and shut down. This is a protective mechanism that is utilized by the body generally under very heavy loads. The novice weightlifter, for example, would have a very low threshold, as his body has not fully adapted to the intramuscular and neuromuscular benefits of weight training. The advanced lifter, through proper training, would have a much higher threshold level than his novice counterpart, allowing him to lift much heavier loads.

Skin receptors can enhance the work of the deeper receptors located in the muscle. Receptors located in the skin of the wrist and fingers can provide information on wrist and finger movements (Lephart et al. 1998).

Other sensors that play a part in the body's ability to function include visual and auditory senses. The ability to see an oncoming potential hit or to hear a warning cue from a helpful teammate allows the body to prepare itself for action. This action may be in the form of muscle contraction and body-segment stabilization, which allow the body to change direction, to absorb the hit efficiently, or to make the play. For example, the hockey player carrying the puck down the ice with his head down is vulnerable to a crushing, open-ice hit. As his teammate yells, "Heads up!" he will instinctively tense up, look around, and prepare his body for a hit.

The Information Pathways

All the information described here is translated for the central nervous system (CNS) by not one specific receptor, but many. The coordinated efforts of all these mechanisms allow our bodies to meet the challenge of functional movement in a changing environment.

The translating receptors send their signals over different pathways to the CNS. Here the signals are broken down and sent to a motor control center, where a decision is made regarding the mechanism of muscle contraction. The resulting contraction is then produced through the use of different motor pathways, thereby transforming neural information into physical energy (Lephart et al. 1998).

The complete function of the nervous system is a complex phenomenon and beyond the scope of this book. The premise is illustrated in figure 1.1.

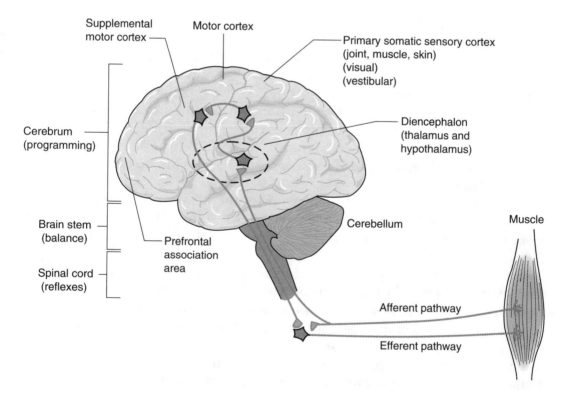

Figure 1.1 Functions of the nervous system.

Addressing deficiencies in the neuromuscular systems described here has been a goal of therapists for many years. One author believes that training to enhance joint muscle receptors should be utilized early in a rehabilitation protocol (Lephart et al. 1997). Activities should focus on sudden alterations in joint positioning that necessitate reflexive neuromuscular control. This type of training utilizes balance and postural activities designed to stimulate muscular coactivation (Lephart et al. 1997). Such coactivation allows for greater loading tasks for the specific joint, which will, in turn, result in larger strength increases and produce a stronger, more functional joint. We have implemented this with our injured athletes to help them recover their dynamic sports athleticism and to help prevent re-injury upon re-entering an unstable competitive environment. Exercises for the hips, back, and shoulder are accurately detailed in this book. The resulting phenomena of increased balance and stability ultimately leads to increased functional strength levels.

Balance

Balance is a state of bodily equilibrium, or the ability to maintain the center of body mass over the base of support without falling (Irrgang et al. 1994). Balance can also be defined in three ways: the ability to maintain a position, the ability to voluntarily move, and the ability to react to a perturbation (Berg 1989). It is quite apparent that all of these definitions are important not only in sport performance, but also in general human movement, which involves challenging balance tasks on a daily basis.

In the body, muscles make up a continuous chain that attempts to overcome disturbances in the center of gravity. The chain begins with the ankle—when there is a challenge of balance that may force the body to lean forward, the muscle in the back of the ankle, the gastrocnemius, will contract to counteract this movement, pulling the body forward in balance. If balance is forced backward, the anterior tibialis muscle will contract and work to pull the body back to its center of gravity.

If the body is supported on only one leg, there is an increased challenge to balance from side to side, which will be counteracted by pronation and supination of the foot at the ankle joint. In some instances, the sway of the body will be too great for the ankle alone to counteract the balance challenge. When this occurs, a person will use the muscles in the legs, hips, and back to counteract the movement.

Remember, your body is a linked system. Each muscle has receptors to assess both its own relative position in space and the body's overall balance. They will effectively communicate with one another, sharing information to try to produce the required movement, since they all have an equally vested interest in the body's performing well and remaining injury-free. This is highly trainable!

Biomechanical Considerations

The biomechanics of movement—both in sport and everyday life—require not only strong abdominal muscles but also a strong, balanced *speed center*. The abdominal muscles, along with the lower back, hip flexors and extensors, adductors and abductors, hip rotators, and glutes, collectively, are identified as the speed center. This name was chosen because, in sport, the listed muscle groups initiate, assist, and stabilize all movement (Twist 2001). A hockey shot, golf swing, football throw, rugby tackle, and tennis serve are all powered by the speed center.

We know of athletes who can bench press 300 pounds forever, but, once they are standing in an erect position, they are easily knocked off balance. That is because they have not incorporated their speed center muscles into their strength development. Functionally, you are only as strong as your weakest link. And the weak link can lead to serious injury.

A scientific study that examined the mechanics of powerlifters' spines during heavy lifting (Cholewicki et al. 1996) found that the lumbar segments L-4 and L-5 of one lifter (who had incurred an injury documented by fluoroscope) reached full flexion. While this happened, the other joints were able to concurrently maintain an angle that prevented full flexion. The authors claimed that this occurred potentially as a result of inappropriate sequencing of muscle forces, or a temporary loss of motor control wisdom. These results prompted a further study (Richardson et al. 1999), which attempted to quantify the stability of the spine through a wide variety of loading tasks. The results of the subsequent study indicated that the occurrence of a motor control error resulting in a temporary reduction in activation to one of the intersegmental muscles could allow rotation at only a single joint, possibly causing passive or other tissue to become irritated or even sustain further damage. The author noted that the greatest risk of this result occurs either when there are high forces in the larger muscles with simultaneous low forces in the small, intersegmental muscles (such as when executing a maximal squat effort) or when all muscle forces are low (such as during a low-level effort) (Richardson et al. 1999).

For athletes preparing for high-force dynamic movement and for fitness enthusiasts who strength train, the intersegmental and stabilizing muscles must be better developed to prevent injury. These intersegmental and stabilizing muscles in the spine, shoulders, hips, knees, and ankles can best be stimulated and overloaded by performing exercises in an unstable environment. This book describes how the stability ball can provide this very environment. It will provide a number of viable options for enhancing an exercise toolkit.

General Points to Consider for All Exercises

Swiss Ball Sizing

Most manufacturers of stability balls make sizing recommendations based on the height of the user. Another general rule states that, when users are seated on the ball, their legs should be parallel to the floor. If the legs are below the parallel level, users will be forced to use poor posture for some exercises.

In many cases, these guidelines are helpful in determining appropriate ball size. As you will see in the exercise descriptions, however, this does not always hold true. There are many examples of exercises that utilize a number of ball sizes as they progress. Optimally, training facilities will have different-sized balls available.

Methods of Progression

There are numerous methods of progressing the level of difficulty when using stability ball exercises. Specific progressions are documented in the text of each exercise, but, as previously stated, your imagination is the only limit to what you can accomplish in exercise development with the stability ball. With this in mind, the following are a few options to consider in progressing your exercises.

1. **Change the base of support.** By decreasing the base of support for an exercise, you can increase the challenge of balance. This can be

(continued)

accomplished by increasing the ball inflation, which will result in a smaller base of support; this can be accomplished by bringing the feet closer together in order to narrow the base of support. Additionally, you can change the base of support by moving from a three-point support to a two-point support. For example, in a push-up position with feet on the ball, attempt to raise one hand off the ground while maintaining position.

2. **Change the length of the lever arm.** As you alter the length of your lever arm from short to long, you increase the difficulty of the exercise. For instance, when using an abdominal crunch medicine ball throw progress by throwing from the chest (short) to throwing from overhead (long).

3. **Increase the range of motion.** Increasing movements from a smaller to a larger range of motion also increases the difficulty of the exercise. When doing push-ups with your hands on the ball, for example, you can progress from partial push-ups to full range. When doing rollouts rolling farther out increases the lever arm and range of motion to add more demands to the core.

4. **Vary the speed of movement.** The challenge of stability within the exercise can be raised by changing the tempo of the exercise. Some exercises, such as medicine ball throws, are more difficult with fast speeds. Other exercises, such as Swiss balls with dual instability are much more difficult when moving slowly.

5. **Add resistance.** You can intensify an exercise by adding some form of resistance, such as an external free weight, a cable, or Spri tubing. Performing the jackknife exercise with a cable attached to the legs is one example.

6. **Close the eyes.** By closing the eyes you increase the proprioceptive demand on the body and introduce a whole new element to any exercise. Use caution here, as proper spotting by a strength coach is necessary for exercises such as kneeling on the ball and closing the eyes.

Setting the Abdominals

Setting the abdominals is a simple, yet important, technique in the setup phase of all stability ball and medicine ball exercises. Slightly drawing in your navel toward your spine and giving your pelvis an anterior tilt (which emphasizes the natural curve in your lower back) accomplishes the setting of the abdominals. This drawing in serves a significant function. Most important, it initiates a support mechanism for the spine and torso as a result of the transversus abdominis and internal oblique muscles being activated. This motion of drawing in has been demonstrated to assist in the reduction of compression on the spine by as much as 40 percent, as well as promoting the natural function of these muscles. When this contraction is activated, it provides your body with a much more stable core area for executing all exercises (Richardson et al. 1999; Wirhed 1990).

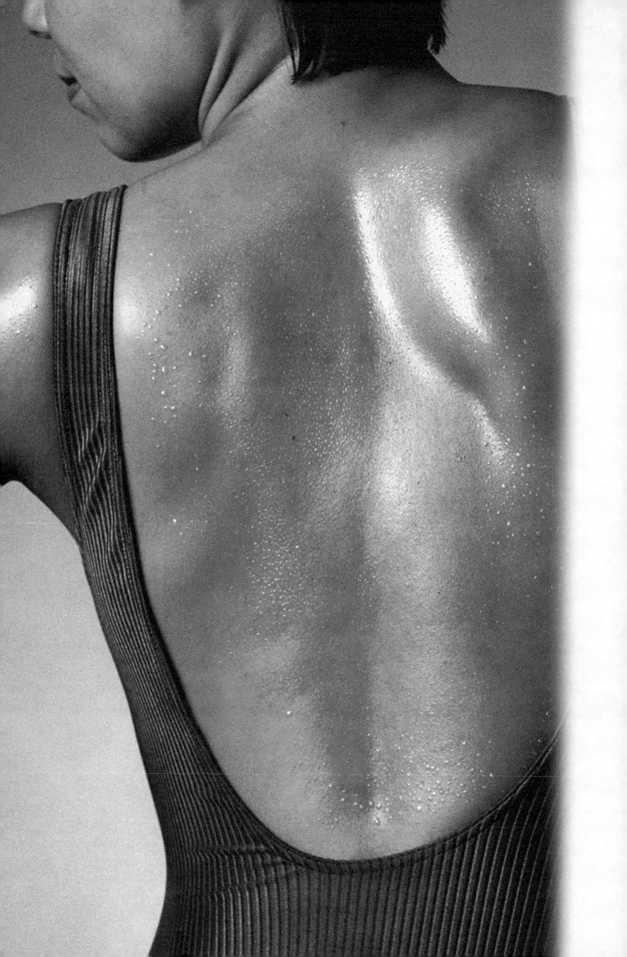

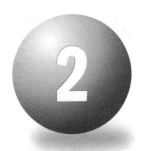

Shoulders and Upper Back

The goal of the prone row external rotation is to integrate two functional movements into one exercise. Recruitment of the spine's extensor muscles is also emphasized during this exercise.

Setup

Place the stability ball under your mid chest, and align your body so that your knees, hips, shoulders, and neck are in a neutral position *(a)*.

Movement

With your hands in an extended position under the shoulders, pull your elbows directly up, ensuring that your upper arms are in a straight line across your body *(b)*. If you were being viewed from the top, it would be possible to draw a straight line from elbow to elbow, right across the upper back *(c)*. The elbows should never rise above this parallel line. Clients with shoulder impingement problems should find a comfortable range of motion slightly below this position, to ease any potential shoulder pain.

Finish

Once you have brought your elbows up, stabilize this position and externally rotate your upper arms. It is important to maintain a 90-degree angle at the elbow joint, as this will guarantee a longer lever, ensuring optimal loading of the external rotator musculature. Rotate until your arm is horizontal to the ground, as demonstrated in the finishing position. Hold this position for one second, and then de-rotate, lowering arms to the initial start position and repeating for the prescribed number of repetitions.

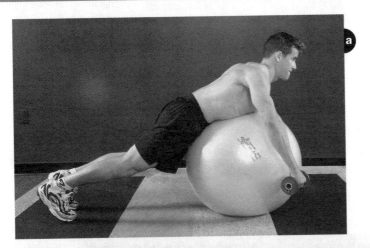

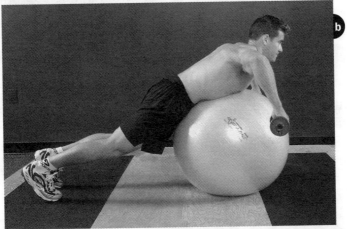

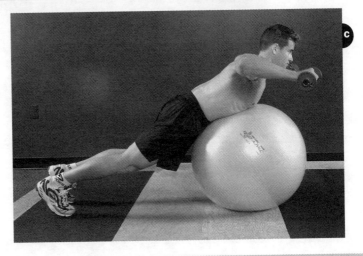

The CBRDR targets the important muscles in the back of the shoulder that help to stabilize the shoulder blade. The position of the body will also challenge your core muscles of the abdomen and back.

Setup

Lie sideways over the ball, with the ball placed in your armpit and to the side of your chest as shown *(a)*. This lateral position must be maintained throughout the movement.

Movement

Begin the movement by setting your abdominal muscles and drawing in your navel. With your arm extended and pointing toward the floor, begin to raise your arm away from your body.

Finish

As you continue to lift your arm, there will be a challenge to your core musculature to stabilize your body on the ball. Continue to maintain good position on the ball. Bring your arm up to a position 5 degrees from perpendicular, as shown *(b)*. Hold this position for two seconds, then lower the weight to the setup position for your next repetition.

Cross Body Rear Delt Raise (CBRDR)

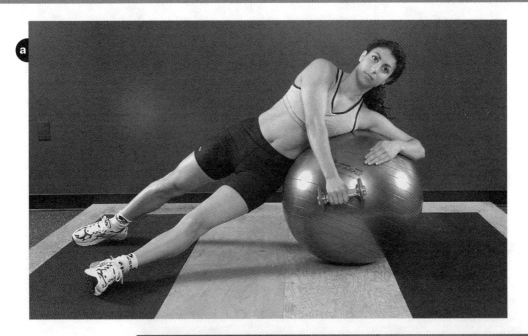

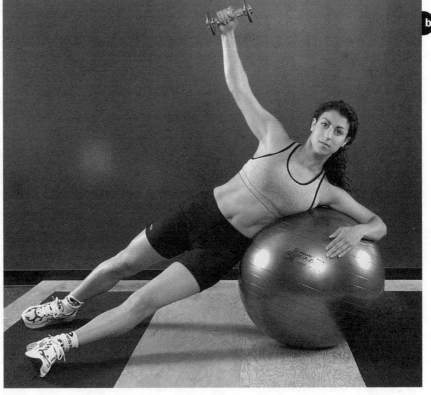

Isodynamic Rear Delt Raise (ISRDR)

The ISRDR is a unique exercise because it incorporates isometric exercise (muscle contraction with no movement) and movement, all in a single drill. The muscles that are targeted here are the muscles that surround the shoulder, shoulder blade, neck extensors, and spine extensors.

Setup

Position for this exercise by lying prone on the ball, with the ball placed just below your chest. Your body should be in a position that aligns the ankles, knees, and hips. The torso should be flexed forward so your upper body is at about a 45-degree angle from the ground. With a dumbbell in each hand maintain the setup position and raise your arms with bent elbows until they are almost parallel to the ground.

Movement

Once your arms are in the proper position (a), there is actually no movement. This is the isometric type of muscle contraction. Hold this position for 5 to 10 seconds. Make sure you maintain good head posture during this effort.

Finish

After 5 to 10 seconds, you will find the shoulder musculature tiring quite quickly. To ease the load, change the angle at which the load is being placed on your shoulders. Bend your knees and roll back on the ball by approximately 20 degrees (b). Maintain the same posture and arm position. You will find that once you have rolled back, you will be able to hold this position for another 5 to 10 seconds. The set is now completed. Lower dumbbells to the floor and rest for the prescribed period of time.

Isodynamic Rear Delt Raise (ISRDR)

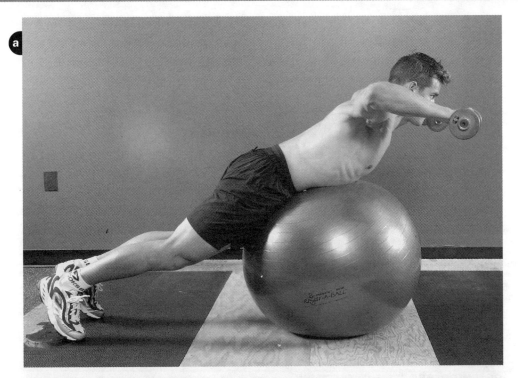

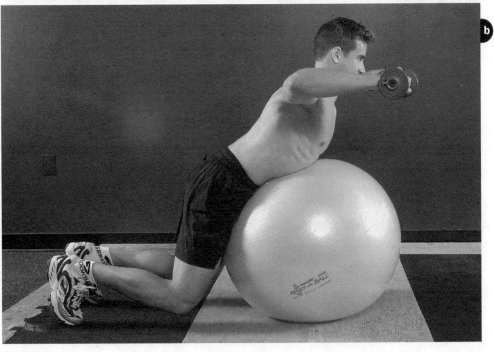

The supine pull-up is a great overall exercise for all muscles in the back side of the body. It requires postural muscles to fire, keeping the body in proper alignment, while the shoulders pull the body up and down.

Setup

You will need to set yourself up in a power rack, so that the height of the barbell will allow for full extension of your arms without your upper back touching the floor. Your grip will determine which muscles will be emphasized *(a)*. An overhand grip, with your elbows pointing outward, will direct more resistance to the posterior deltoid and rhomboids. An underhand grip, with your elbows pointing inward, will emphasize the latissimus dorsi. Hands should be shoulder-width apart or, in the case of the underhand grip, slightly narrower.

Ball placement should begin with the ball under the knees. As you become stronger, you will progress by moving the ball toward your heels. The size of your ball will determine the difficulty of the exercise. Begin with a smaller ball, and again, as you become stronger, progress to a larger ball.

Movement

Before you begin to pull yourself up, it is important to ensure that your knees, hips, and shoulders are aligned. The muscles in your hips and back should be pre-contracted to stabilize your body into this position. Avoid tucking your chin in to view your body. You should be looking at the ceiling, with your head in a neutral position.

As you begin your movement, pull yourself up to touch your chest to the bar *(b)*. As you reach this position, you should attempt to squeeze your shoulder blades together to emphasize the muscles between your shoulder blades and spine.

Finish

As your chest touches the bar, hold this position for two seconds, then lower yourself to the start position. Allow yourself to get a good stretch in your upper back, then repeat.

Supine Pull-Up

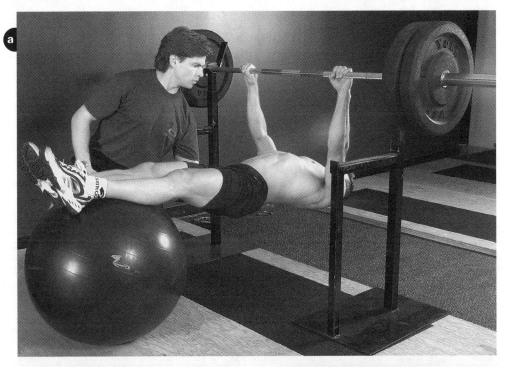

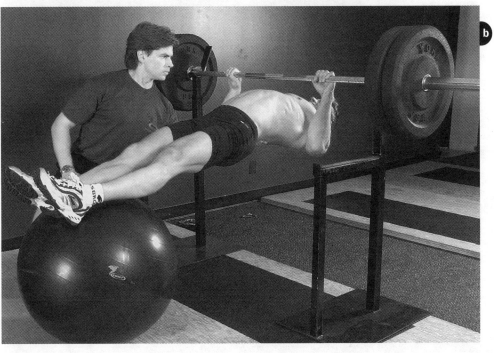

Two very important muscles in the shoulder are the subscapularis and the serratus anterior. These muscles assist in keeping the shoulder blade against the rib cage during arm-pressing movements. Scapular push-ups are an effective method of working this area.

Setup

To set up for the scapular push-up, place your hands approximately shoulder width apart on top of the ball, with your feet back to allow for a 45-degree angle between your body and the floor. Knees, hips, and shoulders should all be in alignment (a).

Movement

The movement is also very similar to that of regular push-ups. The difference is that the elbows do not flex and extend. All movement comes from pushing the shoulder. This pushing movement will create what can be described as a hunched shape of your upper back (b).

Finish

After pushing up until you cannot push any more, slowly lower yourself, allowing your shoulder blades to come together, without bending your elbows.

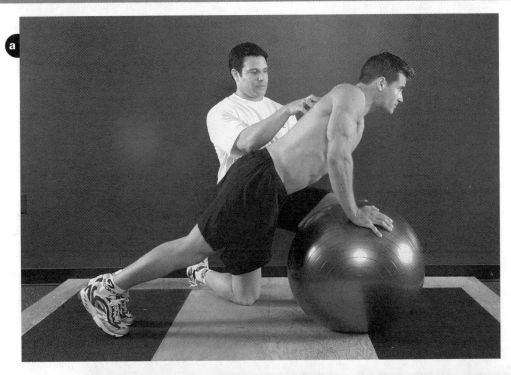

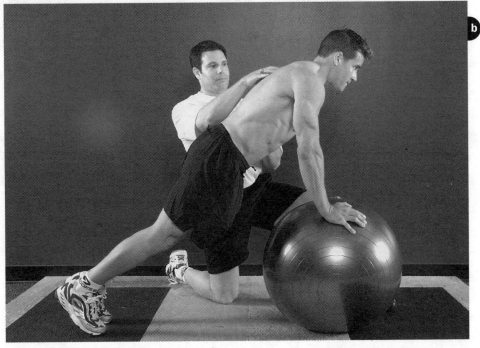

The ability of your muscles to fire powerfully and quickly will generally result in greater protection of your joints. This exercise will train the muscles of the shoulder joint to react very quickly to destabilizing movements from three different positions. The slapping comes from different directions, as well as the shoulder being placed in the positions.

Setup

Sitting on a flat bench, place a ball beside you and extend your arm out to the side, hand on top of the ball. You should be pressing down quite firmly on the ball, not allowing any movement. Ensure that you maintain a straight, tall posture with your chest up, and set your abdominals.

Movement

While you are pressing down on the ball, your partner will begin by slapping the ball in multiple directions with about 60 to 75 percent force. Maximal effort should be given to prevent any kind of movement in the ball. The arm can be held in a position of lateral abduction, or this exercise can be performed with the arm in multiple positions (such as extended in front or at a 45-degree angle).

Finish

The finish will be determined based on the number of ball slaps to be completed. Twenty to thirty rapid ball slaps are recommended.

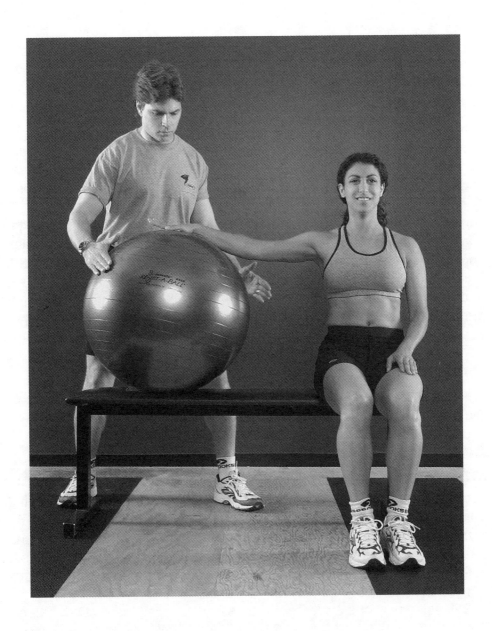

This partner medicine-ball drill develops strength in the shoulder and back region, while working the legs, hips, torso, and upper body.

Setup

Stand facing your partner, about three paces apart. Keep your feet shoulder-width apart, knees slightly flexed, and abdominals pre-contracted.

Movement

Partner A positions his hand and the ball directly in front of his right shoulder (a). The pass line goes from his right shoulder to Partner B's right shoulder. Partner B prepares to receive the ball by flexing her knees, contracting the core, and fully extending her arms, giving her partner a target, cushioning the pass reception with the entire body (b). The ball comes into the hands, the arms bend to draw the ball closer to the right shoulder, the hips drop, and body weight shifts onto the right leg, which should flex at the knee. The pass back reverses the flow by pushing the foot into the ground, extending the leg, rotating with the hip and torso, and extending the arms to thrust the ball back to Partner A. The arm movement is more of a direct push from the shoulder, similar to a shot put throw, rather than a throw one is accustomed to in baseball.

Finish

Continue this sequence for a set number of repetitions. Then repeat the set, throwing from left shoulder to left shoulder.

Advanced Progressions

Execute the same technique and progression with one arm only (c). To catch the ball, you will be more reliant on absorbing and cushioning the ball with your entire body. It becomes a torso and lower-body catch. You are also reliant on the quality of the pass. When first attempting this advanced exercise, your partner will tend to lob a soft, arced pass, which is difficult to catch. A crisp, straight pass from shoulder to shoulder will be easier to cushion and balance.

Still using only one arm, repeat the same exercise instruction, balancing on one leg only. For the right-shoulder-to-right-shoulder partner pass, both partners balance on their left leg. Superior balance, proprioception, core and hip stabilization, and multi-joint pass reception are all challenged.

Medicine Ball Shoulder-to-Shoulder Pass

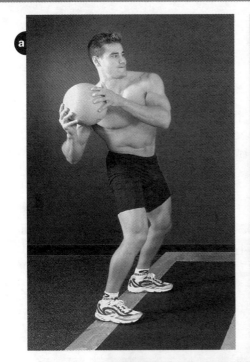
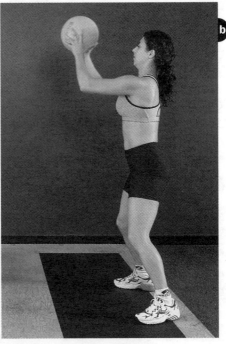

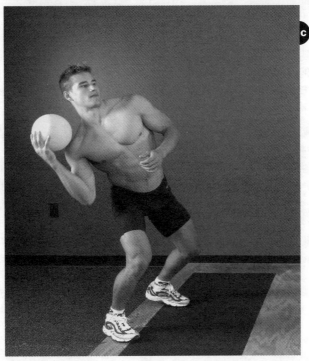

This soccer-specific exercise develops great lat strength and back power for all participants. It expands the torso and requires solid core stability.

Setup

Both partners stand facing each other, about two paces apart. Keep your feet shoulder-width apart, knees slightly flexed, and abdominals pre-contracted. Partner A sets up by holding the ball above her head.

Movement

Partner A begins by dropping the ball behind her head *(a)*, then pulling the ball back over her head until her arms are fully extended. Once the arms are extended and hands are about one foot in front of the body, Partner A will release the ball *(b)*. Pass is aimed above Partner B's head.

Finish

Partner B catches the ball high in the air, about one inch in front of her head. The pass is cushioned by slowing down the ball and progressively absorbing its momentum until it is behind the head. Additional knee flexion during pass reception will help absorb the pass and protect the lower back. Return the pass and continue for desired number of repetitions.

Advanced Progression

Any passes a little too low can be successfully caught by dropping quickly into a squat position, dropping the hips, and flexing the knees as much as needed to catch the ball overhead. We also prescribe this as an advanced progression. The pass can be thrown low, so you squat and catch, and drive up with knee extension on the return pass.

Medicine Ball Soccer Throw-In Pass

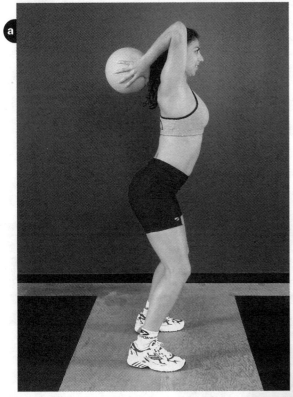

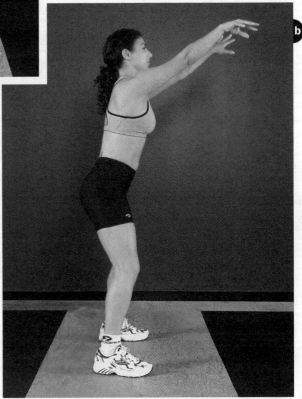

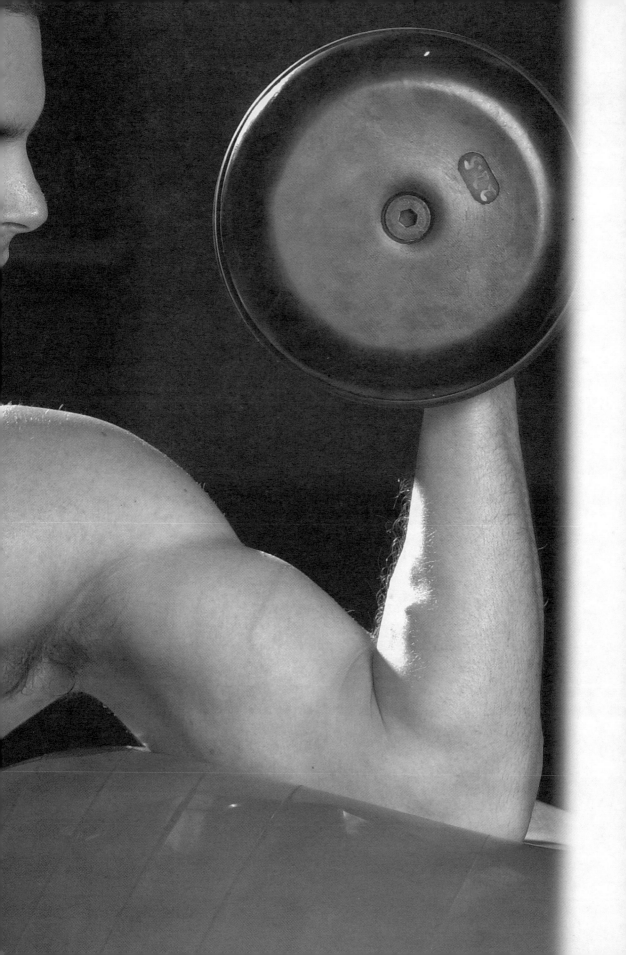

Biceps,
Triceps,
and Forearms

The technique used in this biceps curl provides a means of sensing proper posture and of focusing solely on the movement of the biceps.

Setup

You will need a partner to place the ball between your body and the wall. Ball placement should be just at shoulder-blade level. Stand tall, pressing against the ball, with your chest up and knees slightly bent *(a)*. You should feel the ball against your triceps at all times. This will ensure that you maintain a straight arm position to enhance biceps recruitment.

Movement

While looking straight ahead, pull in your navel, and begin flexing your elbow. Curl the bar until you can flex your arm no further *(b)*.

Finish

Once you have reached the fully flexed position, begin a slow descent back to the starting position. It is important that you lower the weight until your elbow is fully extended.

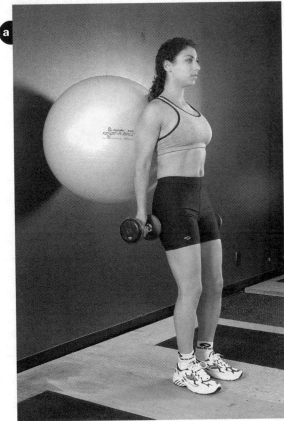

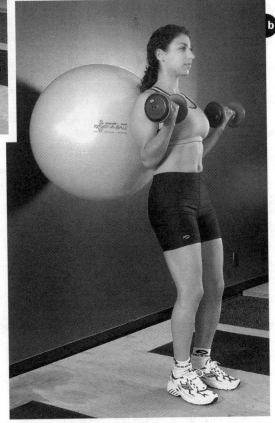

An eccentric contraction occurs when a muscle lengthens under load. Eccentric contractions are known to be significantly stronger than concentric contractions, in which a muscle shortens under load. Therefore, in the biceps curl movement, you can actually lower a heavier weight than you would be able to raise. If you emphasize the eccentric portion of the movement, your potential concentric (or lifting) strength will increase.

Setup

Use a ball size that allows you to lie prone over the ball with your arm fully extended (a). Select a weight that is 20 to 40 percent heavier than you would normally use.

Movement

Because the weight is significantly heavier than you would normally use, to raise it you will have to roll back on the ball (b). This rolling back will provide you with a mechanical advantage to help lift the weight.

Finish

Once you have the weight in a fully flexed position, roll forward again and begin extending your elbow very slowly, returning your upper arm to the downward extended position. It should take you 4 to 6 seconds to lower the weight. Once your arm is fully extended, reposition yourself for the next repetition.

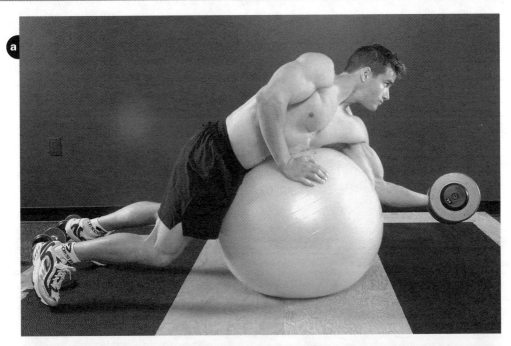

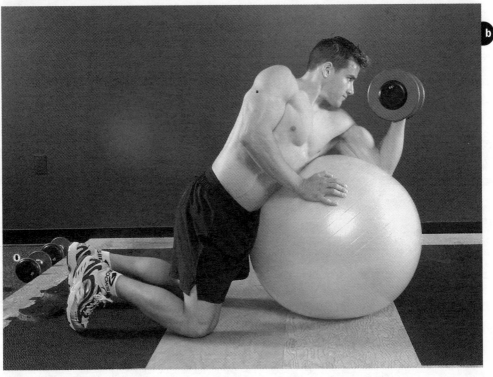

The incline triceps extension will provide a great challenge to the triceps, and, more specifically, to the long head of the triceps. As a result of the overhead position of the arms, the long head will benefit more from this exercise than the other components of the triceps.

Setup

Begin by lying over the Swiss ball on your back. Once in this position, roll forward until the ball is supporting your head, shoulders, and back. Raise your arms overhead in an extended position with dumbbells in hand (a).

Movement

While maintaining an erect upper arm, bend at the elbow joint, lowering the dumbbells until you have reached full elbow flexion (b). At this point, the dumbbells should be on either side of the head.

Finish

To finish this movement, return to the starting position. It is important to keep your elbows pointing straight up as you extend your arms. This will provide optimum isolation for your triceps.

Incline Triceps Extension

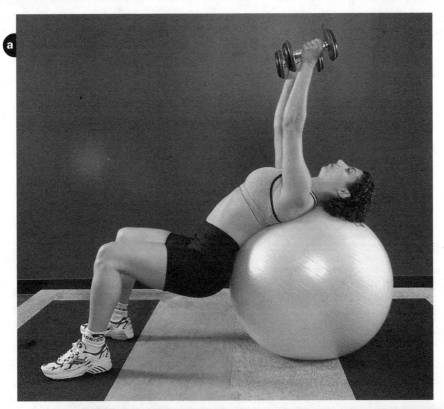

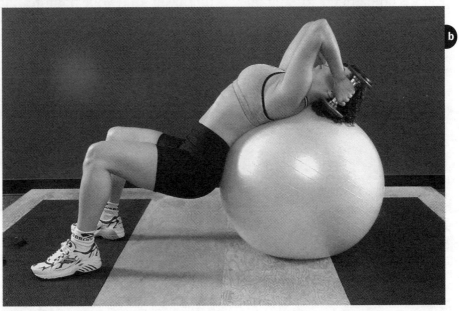

The triceps blaster is an advanced exercise that should only be attempted by the experienced athlete. This exercise should first be attempted with feet on the ground, and, as you become stronger, you can attempt to perform it with feet raised on a bench.

Setup

Place both hands on the ball, with your back in a tight, supported position and your abdominal muscles drawn in *(a)*. Initially, this exercise should be performed with feet on the ground, as previously explained.

Movement

While maintaining your back position and posture, begin by dropping your elbows toward the ground. The movement can be described as wrapping your forearms down and around the ball *(b)*.

Finish

As you reach the bottom position by dropping your elbows, your body will be challenged to stay on the ball. Maintain your posture and extend your arms to bring yourself back to the starting position.

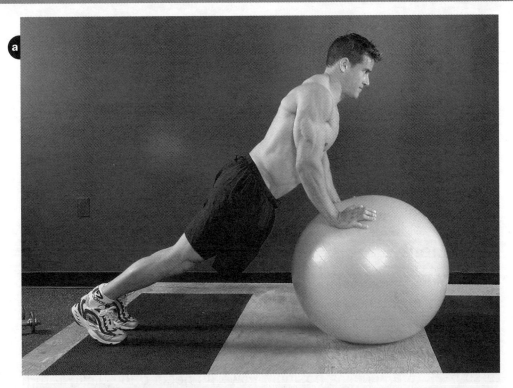

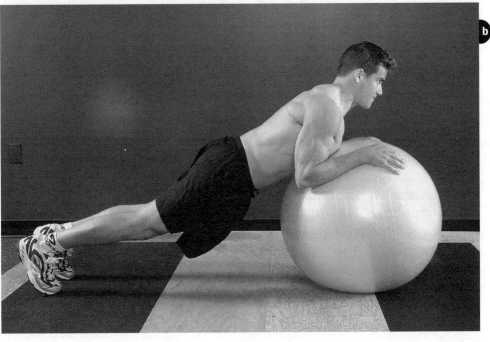

This drill is excellent for improving strength, and endurance in the chest, shoulders, and triceps. It is a great upper-body plyometric exercise because it prepares the body for eccentric loading and concentric power.

Setup

Partners kneel facing each other, two paces apart. Both partners should place their knees on the edge of a stretching mat, keeping most of the mat in front of their bodies. Partner A holds the ball at chest height, with the torso upright.

Movement

Partner A begins by falling forward and forcefully extending the arms to deliver a chest pass to Partner B. After releasing the ball, Partner A will continue to fall until her hands make contact with the mat, absorbing her body into a push-up position (a-c). Immediately and powerfully, Partner A should push back up to reverse the direction and propel the torso back to a kneeling position. Power is needed to quickly return the body to an upright position, ready for a return pass. As soon as both partners are able to make eye contact, Partner B should return the pass in the same manner previously described for Partner A.

Finish

After Partner B has received and returned the chest pass, he should follow through with the same push-up and the same immediate, forceful return to an upright position. Partners should not initiate a throw until eye contact is made, and the partner completing the push-up should focus on being ready to receive the return pass without delay.

Continue this sequence for a set number of repetitions, or until fatigue prevents pushing back up to a kneeling position. Especially as the partners tire, the tempo slows, and decision making is inhibited, remember the importance of waiting for eye contact before returning passes.

Medicine Ball Push-Up and Pass

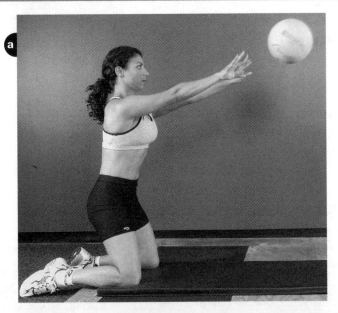

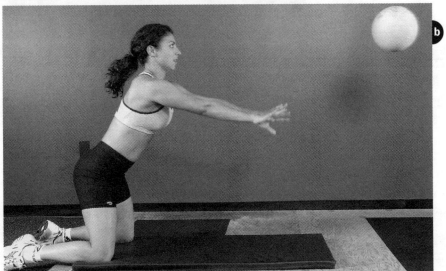

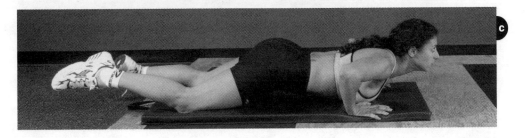

This drill provides a great way to add balance, core stability, and increased strength requirements to the simplicity of executing a push-up.

Setup

Place your body prone, as in a normal push-up position, supported by your hands on the ball and your toes on the ground. Set your abdominals to maintain a strong trunk, creating a straight line from ankles to shoulders. The hands should be placed at 3:00 and 9:00 on the ball. Set your feet together to create a small platform, increasing the balance requirements for the exercise *(a)*.

Movement

While keeping a rigid core, flex the elbows and lower the body with a controlled motion, bringing your chest toward the top of the ball *(b)*.

Finish

Momentarily hold the lowered position, maintaining balance, before extending your arms and returning to a push-up position.

Medicine Ball Push-Up

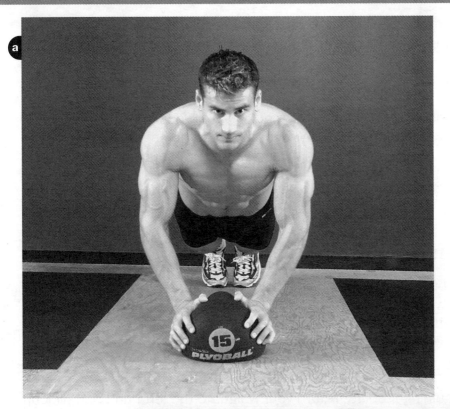

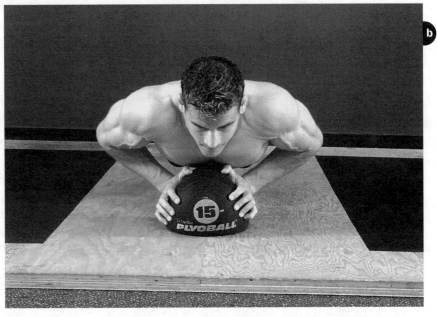

Walk-overs are similar to push-ups, but they activate many more muscles to compensate for uneven surfaces and single-arm loading.

Setup

As described in the setup for medicine ball push-ups, support your body in a prone position with your hands on the ball and your toes on the floor. Again, set your abdominals to maintain a strong trunk. Remove your left hand from the ball and set it on the floor to your left. Keeping your feet in place, shift your upper-body load over your left hand and lower your body with the left arm, as in a regular push-up *(a)*.

Movement

Extend the left arm to push your body up and back over the ball. Transfer your weight to the right hand as you return your left hand from the floor to the ball.

Finish

After regaining stability, return your weight to the left hand and pick up your right hand, placing it on the floor to your right. Next, shift your weight to the right arm and repeat the same push-up motion previously completed *(b-c)*. Continue this sequence until fatigue prevents safe execution.

Advanced Progression

Try a power-over. Power-overs use the same general technique and progression, but they add a plyometric action. When extending the arm to perform the push-up, powerfully drive up to propel the torso into the air. The hand placed on the ball will then leave the ball slightly before the hand placed on the floor has been returned. In the second repetition, when your hand reaches the floor, quickly flex the elbow to drop into a push-up position and immediately explode back up, pushing the torso back up and over the ball. The torso will shift quickly to both the left and right as the hands dance back and forth, executing this drill with speed.

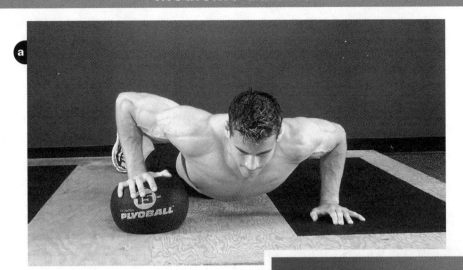

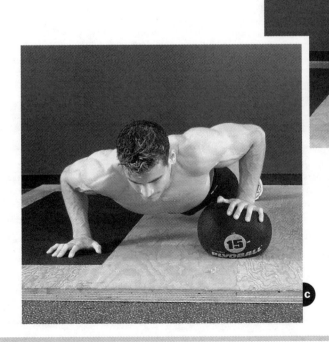

Wrist Curl and Extension

The setup is the same for both wrist curls and wrist extensions. Flexion and extension of the wrist is one area that traditionally has been ignored in strengthening programs. This results from the idea that the wrist muscles receive enough work during other gripping exercises.

Setup

Set up in front of an adjustable cable column. Set the column so that the pulley is approximately 20 degrees below the top of the ball *(a)*.

Movement

Grasping the bar with an underhand grip, begin in the fully extended position and flex your wrists through a full range of movement *(b)*. Hold this position for a second or two.

Finish

Slowly lower the weight back to the original position. For the extension movement, the palms should face the floor.

Wrist Curl and Extension

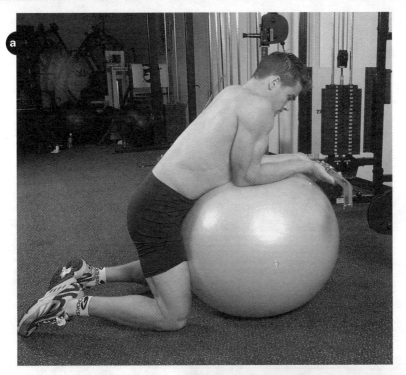

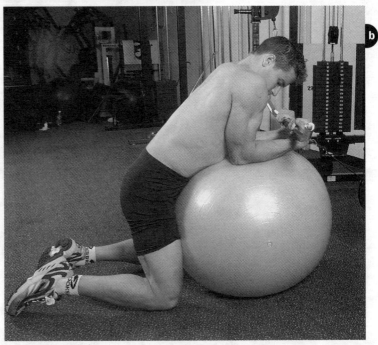

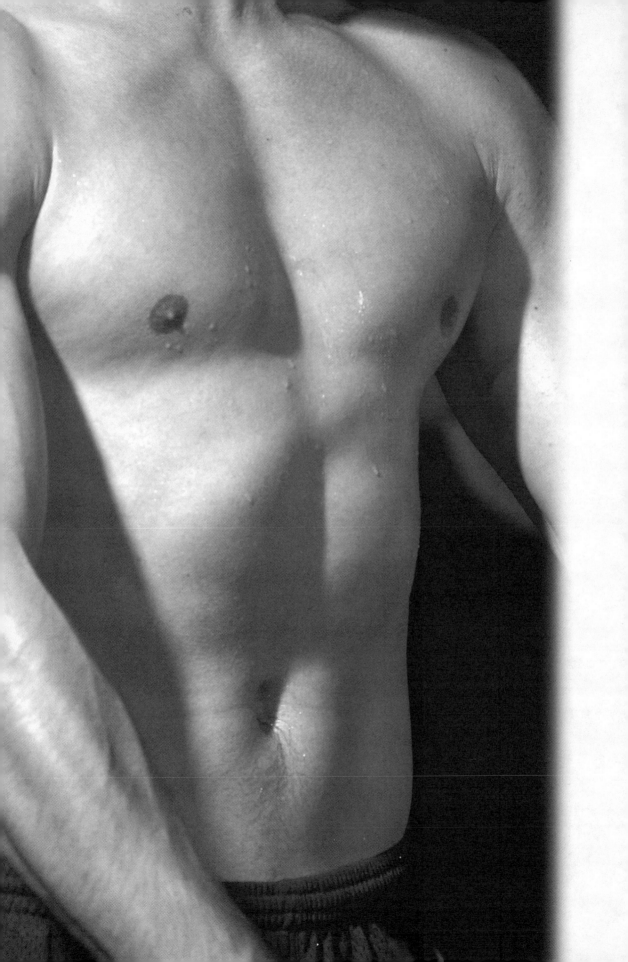

Chest

Focus is on the upper pectoral muscle. This exercise can be performed on a ball, introducing the elements of balance and stability.

Setup

In this exercise a larger ball is necessary for the correct support. Holding the dumbbells that you will be pressing, sit on the ball. Walk slowly out until your head, shoulders, and back are being supported by the ball. To provide a safe initial base of support, be sure to place your feet farther than hip-width apart.

Movement

Begin by setting your abdominals. Press your arms in an upward arc until your hands are above your eyes *(a)*.

Finish

Once you have reached the top position, lower the dumbbells to touch the top of your shoulder *(b)*.

Safety Note: Your floor surface must be clean and free of dust. As you are pressing on the ball at an angle, you need to prevent the ball from rolling out and away from you during the exercise.

Hand Position

The hand position demonstrated here is called the neutral grip position. When the hands are in this position, less stress is placed on the shoulders than in the traditional bench-press position. In the traditional position, the palms are facing away from the body and the shoulders are externally rotated. If you suffer from any kind of shoulder ailment, it is recommended that you utilize the neutral grip position.

Advanced Progressions

Decrease the width of your foot placement. This will increase the challenge for stability in this exercise. Use only a one-arm dumbbell press. This will increase the difficulty of the exercise, and it will require greater core stabilization.

Incline Dumbbell Press

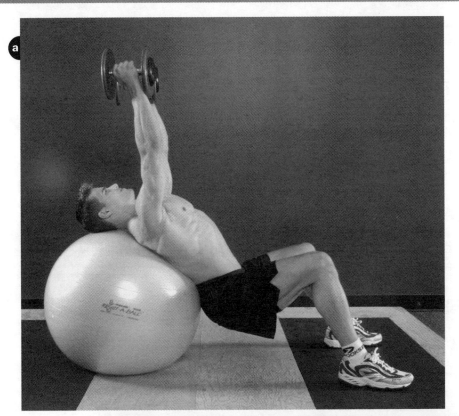

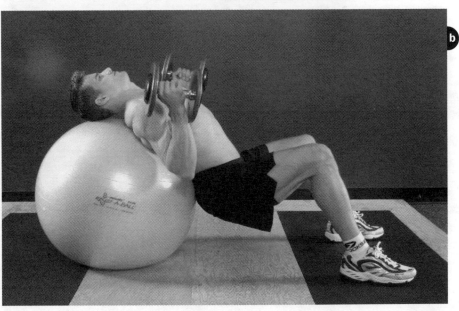

Compared with the previous exercise, this dumbbell press is a more general chest exercise that focuses on the whole pectoral area.

Setup

Hold the dumbbells that you will be pressing. From a seated position on the ball, slowly walk out until your head and shoulders are supported by the ball. Place your feet slightly farther than hip-width apart to provide a safe initial base of support *(a)*.

Movement

Begin by setting your abdominals. Then, press your arms upward until your hands are directly above your eyes *(b)*.

Finish

Once you have reached the top position, move the dumbbells down to rest on your shoulders.

Dumbbell Press

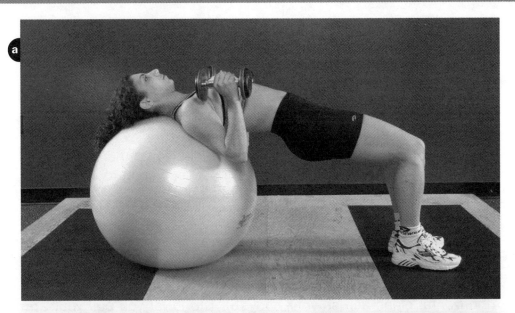

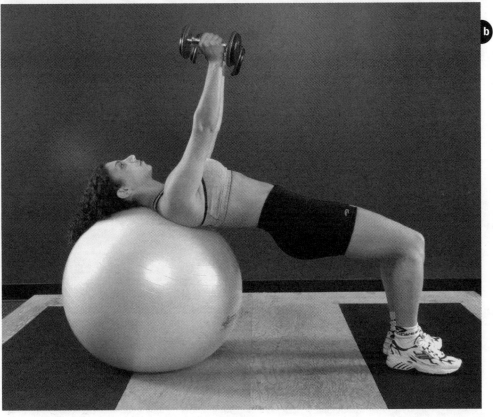

The cable fly provides excellent recruitment of the entire pectoral muscle. Additionally, the single-arm movement makes it extremely demanding for the core musculature to stabilize your body on the ball.

Setup

Place the stability ball beside a low pulley with a single handle attached to the cable. Taking hold of the handle, sit on the ball and roll forward until you are in a supine extended position. Your hips and back should be parallel to the ground (a).

Movement

Your arm should be in the low position, with the elbow slightly bent. This will alleviate any stress at the elbow joint. Movement should be in a horizontal plane across your body (b). The lower you pull your arm across, the more activation the sternal portion of your pectoral muscle will receive. The higher you pull, the greater the activation of the clavicular part of the muscle.

Finish

Move your arm completely through your range of motion. Hold the final position for one second, and then return to the initial position.

Cable Fly

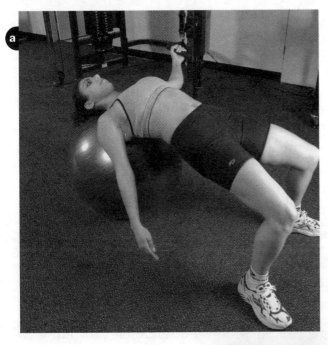

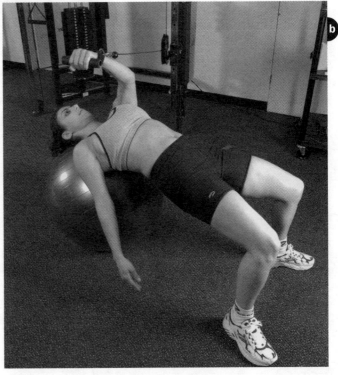

The dual-ball fly is the perfect replacement for the pec deck. The pec deck is sometimes referred to a pec fly machine. This may be a more appropriate term. Not only will you get to work your chest in a very demanding exercise, you also work your entire body as you attempt to maintain proper posture. However, those who have any type of shoulder problem should avoid this exercise, as it places great stress on the anterior capsule of the shoulder.

Setup

You will need to use two stability balls. Bring both balls together, side by side. Place one of your lower arms on each ball. Your body should be approximately at a 45-degree angle with normal curvature of your low back *(a)*.

Movement

Begin movement by rolling the balls outward, allowing your arms to open up. Continue until you feel you have reached a comfortable range of motion *(b)*.

Finish

Once you have reached the range of movement you are comfortable with, squeeze your arms back together, bringing the balls back to their original position.

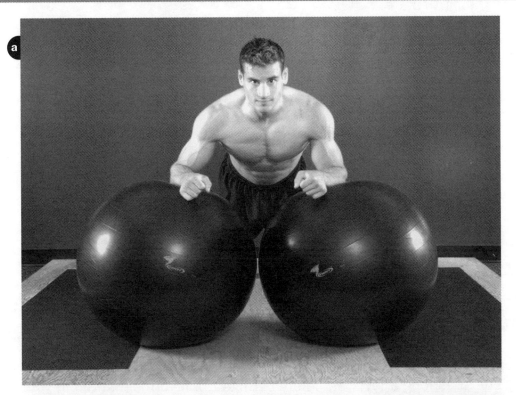

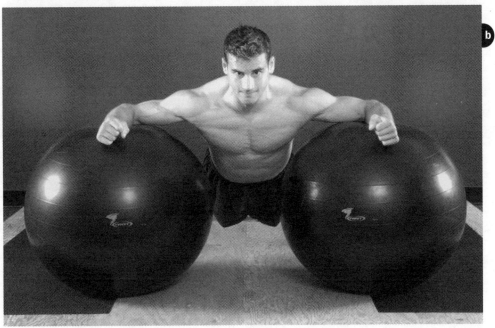

This exercise places the body in a closed kinetic chain athletic stance. An aggressive abdominal and low back exercise, the standing two-ball roll-out also requires contribution from all major muscle groups in the body, from foot to fingertip, as an ultimate, linked system. Development of the entire shoulder girdle is also emphasized.

Setup

Stand in front of two balls positioned side by side. Move your glutes forward, and draw in your navel toward your spine to create a pelvic tilt. Keeping your torso upright, flex at your knees and drop your hips into a balanced athletic stance. Place one hand atop each ball, shifting some of your weight to your hands. The load should be distributed equally between your legs, upper body, and core *(a)*.

Movement

Keeping your hands in place, pivot on your toes as you roll the balls away from your body. To maintain equal load distribution throughout your body, drop your hips as the ball rolls away from your knees. Roll out to as long a lever as safety permits *(b)*. If you feel strain in your lower back, make sure you do not allow your back to hyperextend and only roll out to a position that is comfortable. Pelvic position is key here.

Finish

At the farthest reach, hold your position for two seconds. Then, roll back to the starting position.

Advanced Progression

Advance this exercise using alternate rolls. Follow the setup instructions previously given. Then, keeping your hands in place, pivot on your toes as you roll the balls away from your body. Shift your weight up and over both balls to achieve a push-up position atop the balls. This is your starting position. Holding your feet, legs, and hips in place, concurrently roll one ball back in toward your body and the other farther away. Continue in this pattern for the designated number of repetitions.

Standing Two-Ball Roll-Out

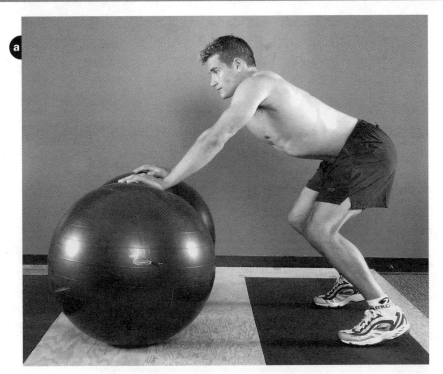

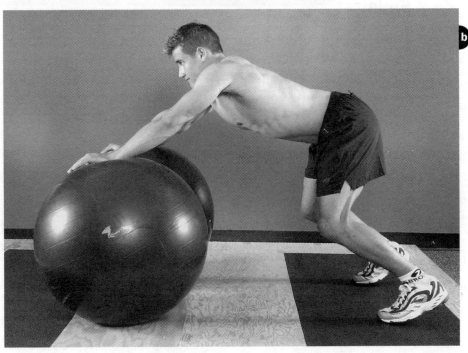

Walk-Out Into Push-Up

This exercise challenges the upper-body musculature while still requiring core strength and stabilization. This is an excellent shoulder stabilization exercise because it stimulates the posterior deltoids.

Setup

From a standing position behind the ball, crouch down, place your abdomen on top of the ball, and roll forward until your hands reach the ground. Walk out with your hands until the ball has rolled past your hips and is under your quadriceps *(a)*.

Movement

At this point it is important to maintain a strong core, contracting the postural muscles to keep the hips up and the body aligned. In other words, focus on preventing your hips from sagging, and avoid any hip or torso rotation. Continue to walk out with your hands until only your feet remain atop the ball *(b)*.

Finish

Complete the movement by doing one push-up, and then walk your hands back in toward the ball until your hips are once again atop the ball. Pay close attention to the movement of your shoulder blade. If, as you lower yourself, your shoulder blade is winging or protruding, you should avoid this exercise and seek medical advice.

Advanced Progressions

When you complete the push-up, hold only one foot atop the ball. Remove the other leg at the far position of each repetition and hold it straight. Walk out as quickly as you can. Then, to return back to the ball, jump with both hands together in a plyometric action, shuffling back to the setup position.

Walk out as slowly as you can, extending the time your body is supported by only one hand. Be sure to keep your hips up, strong and aligned, without hip or torso rotation—your shoulders and hips should face square to the ground.

Walk-Out Into Push-Up

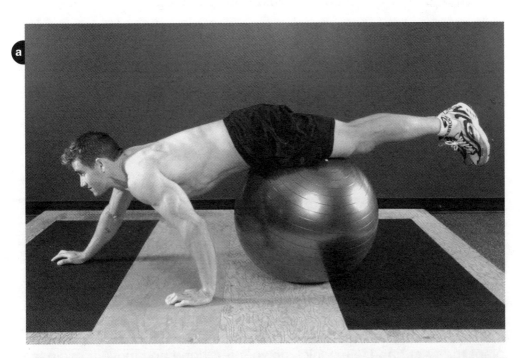

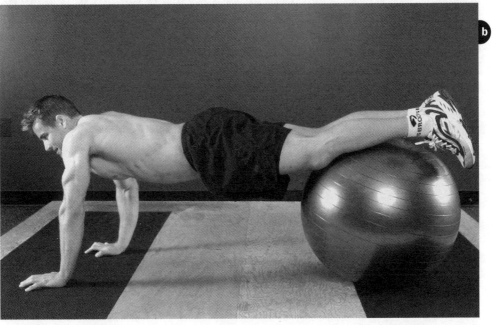

This is a great exercise for shoulder stabilization and core stability. The purpose is to load each shoulder independently.

Setup

From a standing position, crouch down and rest your abdomen on top of the ball in front of you. Roll forward until your hands reach the ground in front of the ball. Walk out with your hands until only your feet remain on the ball *(a)*.

Movement

At this point it is important to focus on maintaining a strong core, contracting the postural muscles to keep the hips up and body aligned. As in the previous exercise, you should prevent your hips from sagging and avoid any hip or torso rotation. Keep your feet on the ball, with the body in a push-up position to maintain a long lever. Begin to walk your hands laterally, rotating your body around the ball in a clockwise direction *(b)*. To do this, pick up your right hand and move it away from your midline, supporting your body weight with your left arm until you replant the right hand. Next, pick up your left hand and move it in closer to the right hand. Alternate these steps so that your hands will complete a circle around the ball. Maintain a strong body alignment as you move your hands.

Finish

The movement is completed once you have rotated 360 degrees. To repeat this exercise, perform the same movement in a counterclockwise direction.

Ball Walk-Around

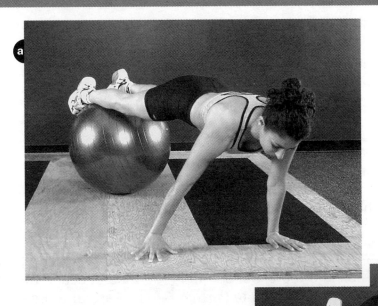

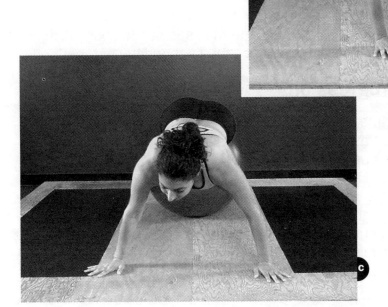

Chest passes link strength and power in the muscles of the chest, shoulders, and back. The catch is absorbed with the core and legs. The return pass is initiated from the legs and hips, and completed with the chest and arms.

Setup

Stand facing your partner, about three paces apart. Keep your feet shoulder-width apart, knees slightly flexed, and abdominals pre-contracted. Both participants should fully extend their arms, in a position level with the chest. Open your hands to make a definitive target.

Movement

Partner A draws the ball into the chest and then reverses direction to push the ball out away from the body to Partner B *(a-b)*. Partner B first makes ball contact with her arms fully extended. The ball is sequentially absorbed by flexing the arms and knees to cushion the catch. Partner B tries to overcome the eccentric loading as quickly as possible, immediately reversing direction to push the ball back toward Partner A.

Finish

After the pass, keep your arms fully extended and hands open, as in the setup position. Continue this sequence for a set number of repetitions.

Advanced Progressions

Complete the same exercise technique, but this time position only two paces apart. Pass as quickly as possible, trying to eliminate any pause at the chest between the negative and positive phases of movement. Hand targets are very important here, both to protect your face and to maintain the rapid pass succession.

To increase strength, repeat the same exercise instruction, five paces apart. You should still attempt to minimize the time between the negative and the positive phase. However, the load you catch will be heavier with the extra distance. More full-body, linked strength is needed to propel the ball the required distance.

Medicine Ball Chest Pass

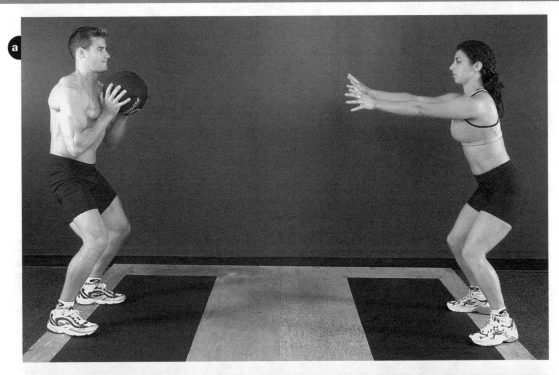

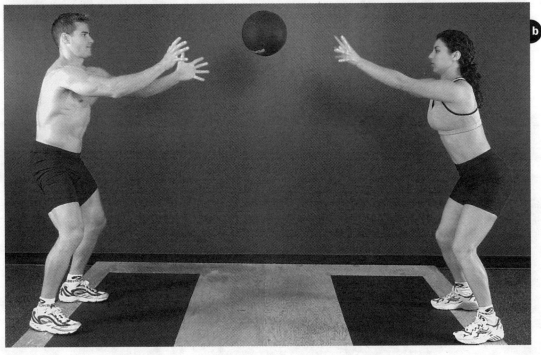

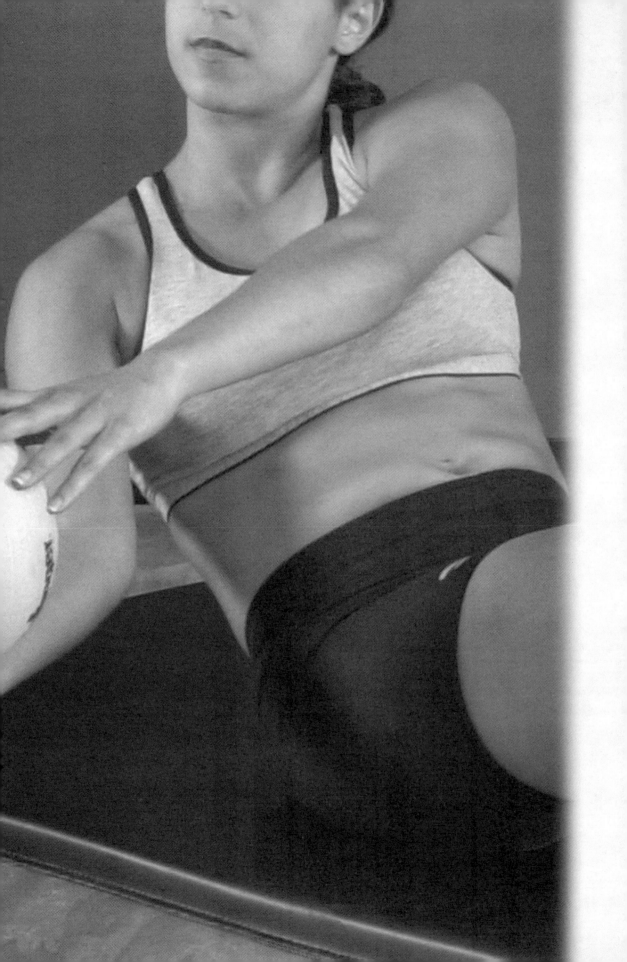

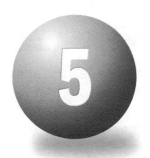

Core Stabilization

To shift the load to your lower abdominal muscles and hip flexors, add this exercise to your program. It requires upper-body and core stabilization, and it activates the lower abs and hip muscles to draw the ball in toward the body. Your lower-body weight is transferred through the ball to produce a load against the hip flexors.

Setup

Standing behind the ball, crouch down and place your abdomen on top of the ball. Roll forward until your hands reach the ground in front of the ball. Walk your hands out until only your feet remain atop the ball. Contract the core to hold a strong link—your body should be in a straight, firm line from head to foot *(a)*.

Movement

Hold your push-up position and retain a strong core. Keep your torso facing square to the ground. Bend at the knees and pull the ball up toward your torso, as if to draw your knees in to your chest *(b)*. Keep the speed of movement under control, with a 1:1:1 tempo.

Finish

Extend your legs to move the ball back to the start position. At the end of each repetition, your body should be linked by strong contractions forming one level, straight line.

Advanced Progression

Follow the same exercise instructions, but work one leg at a time. Begin with only your left foot on the ball. Your right leg should be off the ball, yet straight and firm. Draw the ball up toward your chest with your lower abdominal muscles and hip flexors. Balance on the one leg in this position, holding your contraction, before straightening the left leg back to the setup position, following a 1:2:1 tempo.

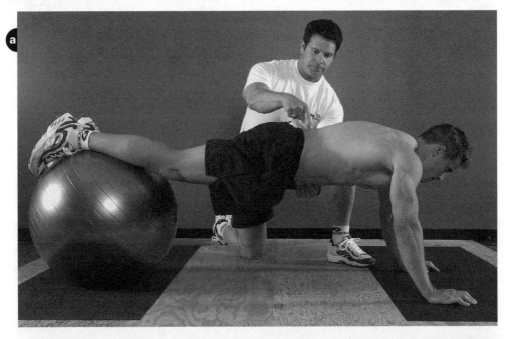

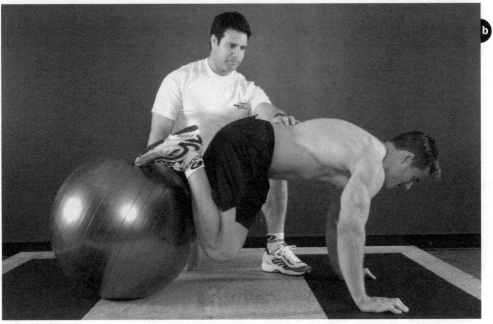

The bridge is a key position that dozens of exercises build on. Bridge fall-offs activate the deep abdominal wall muscles and all core muscles in order to hold the bridge, brake before falling, and pull back into position. This exercise works muscles on every side of the torso.

Setup

Sit atop the ball. Slowly roll forward, leaning back as you roll, until your hips move off the ball. Continue until your middle back is atop the ball. You will feel your shoulder blades at the top and middle of the ball. Place your feet flat on the ground and shoulder-width apart, with your upper legs parallel to the ground. The key to a functional bridge is to elevate your hips, forming a straight line from neck to knees. Be sure your hips are in this position. Next, raise your arms out to the side so that your torso and arms form a T *(a)*.

Movement

Slowly shift your weight to one side, rolling out onto your triceps. Keep your hips up, not allowing any rotation at the hips or shoulders. Move as far to the side as you can without losing your solid position and without falling off the ball *(b)*.

Finish

Using your core muscles, pull your body back across the ball until your shoulder blades are back to the setup position. Continue to move through to the opposite side and repeat movement.

Spotting Tip

Place a dowel across the chest from shoulder to shoulder to evaluate stability and body alignment. Any hip or torso rotation will be evident if the dowel rolls, tips, or falls off.

Advanced Progression

Successful execution of bridge fall-offs can lead to reaction fall-offs. As a partner lightly pushes you to the left or the right, decelerate the movement with your core muscles, reversing your movement to prevent falling off the ball. This is more sport-like, because the main concern is to produce the resultant function rather than to emphasize a strict technique. When pushed to the extreme side ranges, you will tend to roll your torso before braking and returning to your middle setup position.

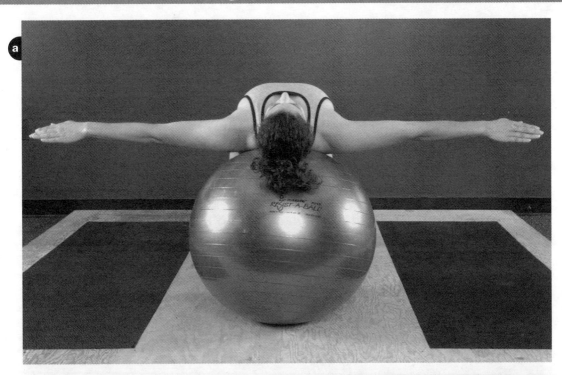

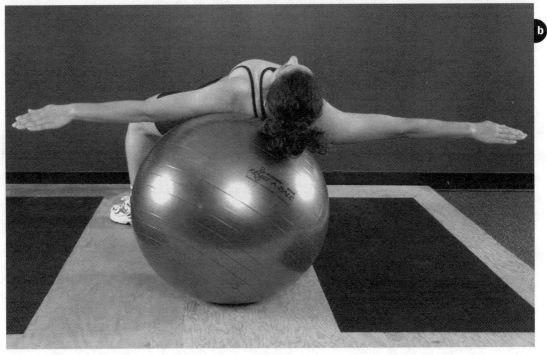

This exercise requires the core muscles to eccentrically decelerate the falling load provided by the medicine ball. In addition, these muscles must produce stabilization, both to hold the basic bridge and to return to balance after catching the ball.

Setup

Sit atop the ball and, while leaning back, slowly roll forward until your middle back is atop the ball. As described in the previous exercise, your shoulder blades should be at the top and middle of the ball, your feet placed shoulder-width apart on the ground, and your upper legs parallel to the ground. Hold your hips up to form a straight line from neck to knees. Extend your arms up above your chest, with your hands in a catching position (a).

Movement

Your partner will stand in front of you and lightly toss a medicine ball so it drops outside your center of gravity. You must rotate slightly to catch the ball as it drops to the right or left of your chest area. Maintain an elevated hip position as you catch the ball (b).

Finish

Brake, balance, and throw the ball back to your partner before using your core to return to the setup position. Continue for the desired number of repetitions.

Spotting Tips

Randomize the medicine ball tosses from left to right, above the shoulder to waist level, as well as overhead. Let the spotter know if you can handle more challenging drops. Also, your spotter should remind you to keep your hips up and to bring your feet back to the starting stance. Without this type of feedback, you may automatically widen your stance when catching the ball, rather than relying on your core strength.

Advanced Progression

Perform the same exercise with your feet right together, rather than using a shoulder-width stance.

Bridge With Medicine Ball Drop

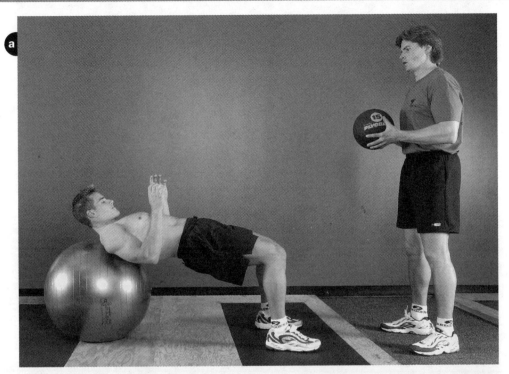

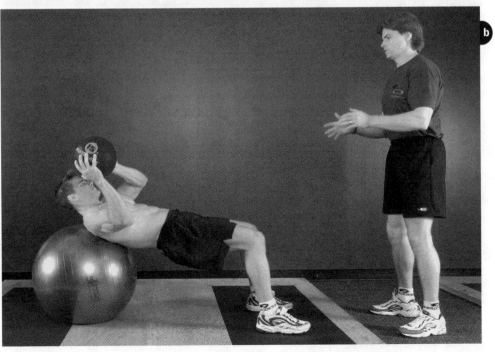

The bridge ball-hug will introduce the concept of static and dynamic contractions to the same exercise.

Setup

As in the previous exercises, sit atop the ball and slowly roll forward to attain the bridge position. Ensure that your middle back is atop the ball, your shoulder blades are at the top and middle of the ball, and your feet are flat on the ground in a shoulder-width stance. Your hips should be elevated to form a straight line from neck to knees, with your upper legs parallel to the ground. Place another ball on your chest, wrapping your arms around as if you were hugging the ball *(a)*.

Movement

Maintain your setup position, and have a partner begin slapping the ball at multiple angles *(b)*. The key is to hug the ball as tightly as possible, limiting the movement of your body and the ball during the slaps. Setting your abdominals during this exercise will assist in stabilizing your body.

Finish

This exercise is completed when the total number of slaps in a set has been reached. The recommended number is 20 to 30 slaps.

Advanced Progression

You can increase the difficulty of this exercise by holding the ball away from your body, with arms extended over your chest.

Bridge Ball-Hug

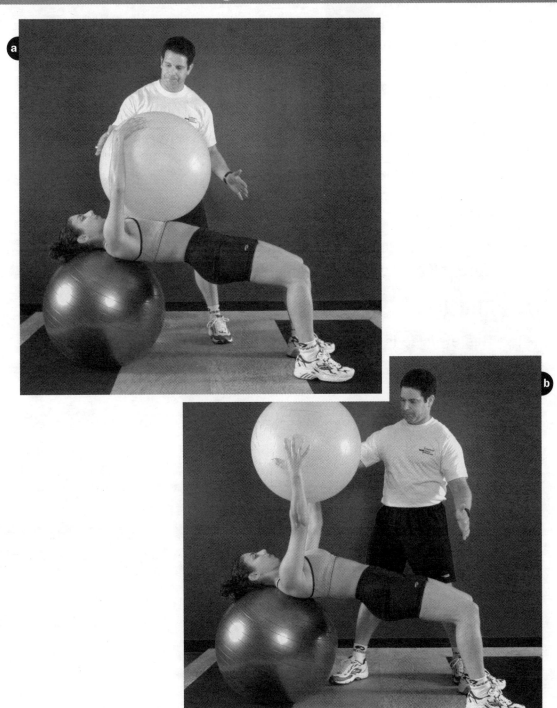

The standing ball-hug is a progression from the bridge position. The standing position is the most sport-specific position you can be in.

Setup

Place your feet shoulder-width apart, with your hips back and your shoulders forward over your knees. This is a very athletic position, and should be maintained for the entirety of this exercise. In this position, hug the ball at torso level.

Movement

Your partner will begin by slapping the ball in multiple directions, as you attempt to maintain your setup position.

Finish

This exercise is completed when the total number of slaps in a set has been reached. The recommended number is 20 to 30 slaps.

Standing Ball-Hug

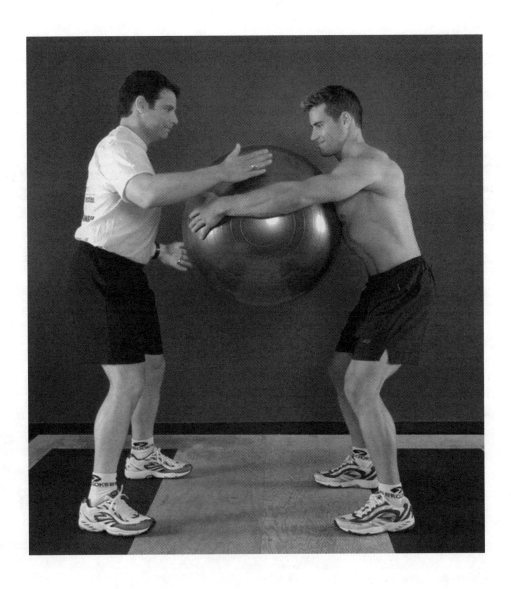

This exercise activates all of the upper-body and core muscle groups for stabilization throughout the exercise. It is a great way to overload the muscles without loading up Olympic weights.

Setup

Standing behind the ball, place your hands shoulder-width apart on the ball. Shuffle your feet back until your chest is over the ball and your toes touch the ground (a).

Movement

Slowly bend your elbows to a 90-degree angle, lowering your chest to the ball. Maintain a strongly contracted core—do not let your hips relax and sag. Hold the lowered position for two seconds, keeping your shoulders and hips square (b).

Finish

Extend your arms to bring your upper body back to the setup position.

Advanced Progressions

In the push-up position, lift one foot off the ground and work to balance as you lower and push up. At the setup stage, place your hands on the sides of the ball rather than on top. Press into the ball as you lower and raise your body.

Balance Push-Up

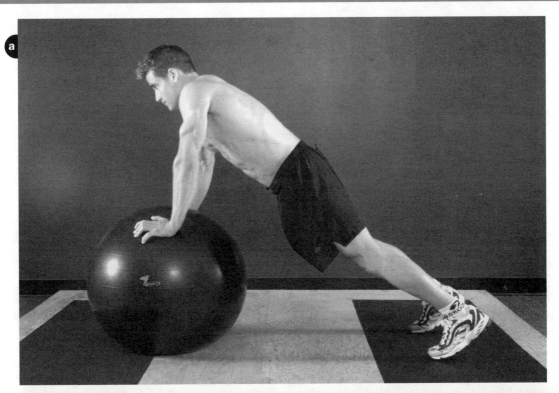

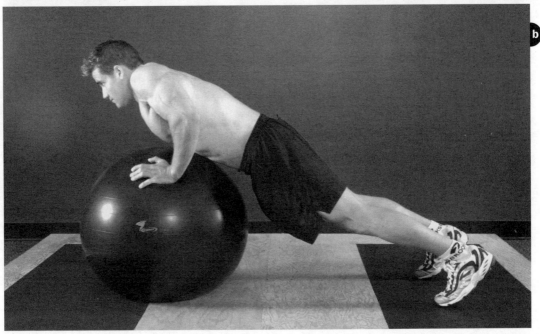

An elevated foot placement moves more of the load to your upper body, and requires more core and hip stabilization. We recommend this exercise in combination with balance push-ups.

Setup

Standing behind the ball, crouch down and place your abdomen on top of the ball. As with the jackknife, roll forward to a push-up position, with your hands on the ground and only your feet atop the ball. Contract the core to hold your body in a straight line from head to foot.

Movement

As you bend at the elbows to lower your chest to the ground, maintain your balance on the ball. Keep your torso facing square to the ground

Finish

Hold your lowered position for one second, then extend your arms to bring your upper body back to the setup position.

Advanced Progression

Once in the setup position, have a spotter position a balance board to produce dual instability. As you lower into the push-up, you must keep your arms balanced on the board as well as your feet balanced on the ball (a-b). Your core must be strongly contracted to link the body together from these two unstable positions.

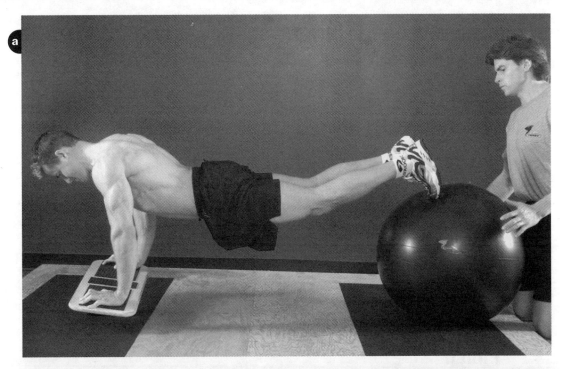

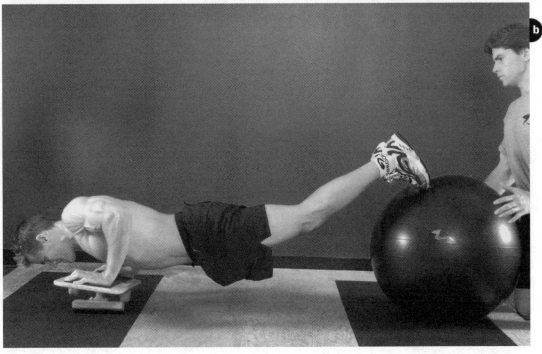

Kneeling on the ball is an excellent method of teaching balance and coordination to an athlete of any age. It requires all the muscles in your core to work together to obtain balance on the ball.

Setup

Begin by placing the stability ball close to a sturdy piece of equipment that you can hold on to if necessary. Place the ball in front of you and kneel over the ball. You will need to hold on to something solid as you get into the actual on-ball position. Make sure that your abdominals are set, and attempt to be as tall as possible.

Movement

If you perform this exercise perfectly, there will be no movement. Therefore, that should be your goal. Maintain as straight a body position as possible without falling off the ball.

Finish

The exercise is completed after you have attempted to stay on the ball for the allotted time. In many cases we have worked with sets of 40- to 180-second attempts. If you fall off the ball, get back on until your set time is completed.

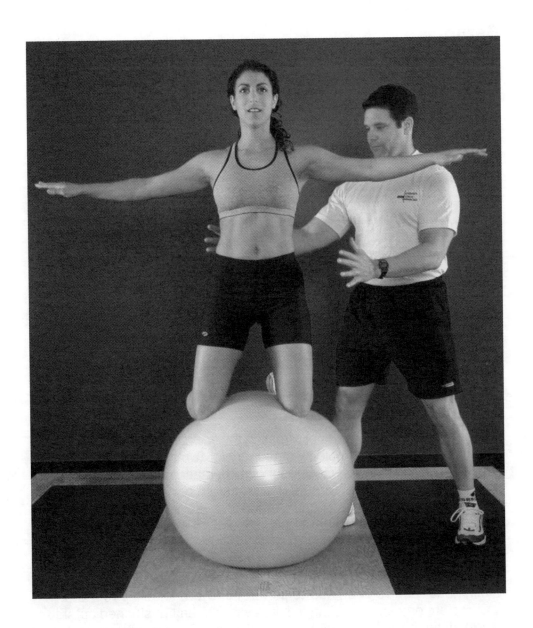

This exercise uses a natural rolling motion to overload the core through a full range of movement producing eccentric elongation as well as isometric contraction.

Setup

Kneel in front of a ball. Move your glutes forward and draw your navel in toward your spine, producing a pelvic tilt. Place your hands atop the ball and bring your feet off the ground. This allows your knees to become the pivot point. Walk your hands out on the ball, moving both the ball and your arms away from your body *(a)*. Once you feel your abdominal muscles beginning to work, you have established your starting position.

Movement

Now your hands should remain stationary on the ball. Pivot on your knees, bringing your torso and hips forward as the ball rolls away from your knees. Keep moving until your chest drops down. Try to keep your chest as upright as possible, without hyperextending your lower back. Keep a neutral spine position as pictured *(b)*. If you feel any strain in your lower back, make sure you are not positioned incorrectly or return to the setup stage and check your pelvic tilt.

Finish

Hold your position at the far reach for two seconds. Then, roll back to the starting position.

Advanced Progressions

There are a variety of ways to progress in this exercise. In the extended roll-out position, rather than holding stationary for two seconds, move the ball outside of your midline to place additional demands on the core muscles. Try a figure-eight pattern, a side-to-side movement aimed at moving the right hand in front of the left shoulder and then reversing the movement. Or, select a word to spell. For example, choose "power," and, in the far extended position, move the ball to spell each letter in "power." One repetition consists of completing the word before returning to the setup position.

Progress to a single-arm roll-out. Keep the ball positioned down your midline and remove one hand to perform one-arm kneeling roll-outs.

Complete one-arm kneeling roll-outs with the ball positioned outside of your midline, more in line with your active arm. This produces additional loading on the shoulder, triceps, and abdominal musculature. Stabilizing muscles have to work harder to prevent hip and torso rotation.

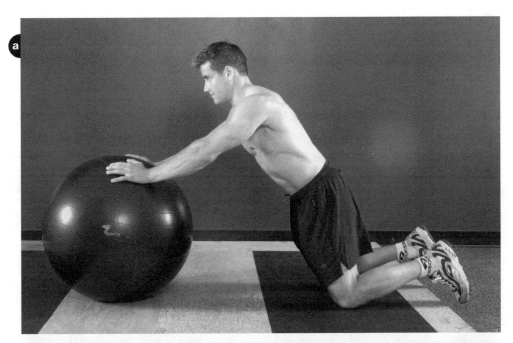

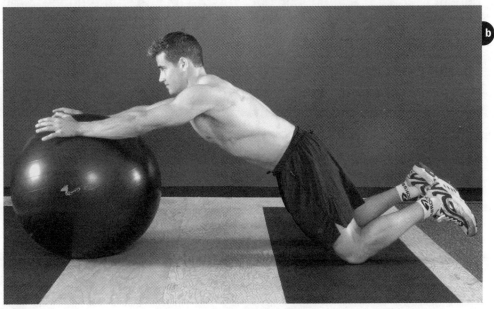

This is one of the best exercises for overloading the abdominal muscles, yet the easiest for maintaining a straight back.

Setup

Set a multi-bench at a 30-degree angle. Standing in front of the bench, set the ball on the seat. Position yourself on your toes, with knees flexed and abdominals set.

Movement

Place your hands on the ball and roll the ball up the bench incline, pivoting forward on the toes *(a)*.

Finish

Roll back down the bench to the start position *(b)*.

Advanced Progression

Stand at the back of the bench. Position the ball at the top of the bench. Using the same technique, roll the ball down the bench. Stop at the end of your range of motion and use your abdominal muscles to pull the ball back up the bench until you are standing upright.

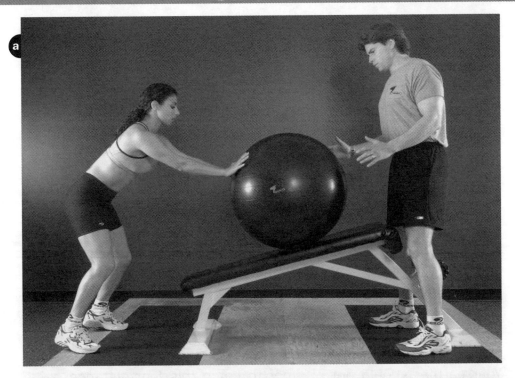

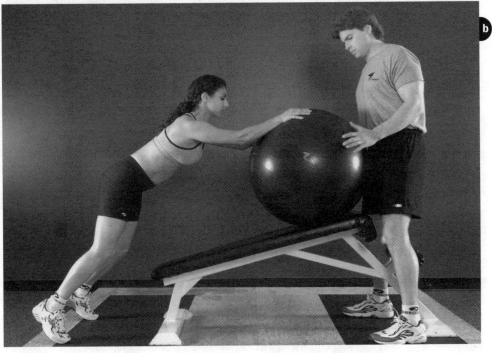

Full-Body Multi-Joint Medicine Ball Pass

This exercise produces sequential, full-body power as well as anaerobic conditioning.

Setup

Stand facing your partner, about six paces apart. Keep your feet shoulder-width apart, your knees slightly flexed, and your abdominals pre-contracted.

Movement

Before you pass the ball, squat down and touch the ball to the floor. Be careful to maintain a good squat position, with the chest safely up and back *(a)*. The throw begins with the legs, transfers through the hips, and moves on to the upper body. Jump off the ground to finish the pass with a powerful leg extension *(b)*. The force-ground relationship is important here. The desired ball direction is forward, not just up.

Finish

Your partner should not attempt to catch this long-distance pass. Through trial and error, your partner will be able to attain a position that allows the ball to land on the ground. The ball can then be caught as it bounces, which is safer and easier on the body. After receiving the ball, your partner squats, touching the ball to the ground, before driving up and forward with the entire body to return the pass at a maximal distance. Every pass should be your best effort.

Advanced Progression

To increase the difficulty of this exercise, attempt a Get-Twisted, lateral two-ball pass. This drill uses the same throw technique. Both partners start with a medicine ball at opposite sides of the drill course. On the signal, both throw for maximal distance, then immediately begin a quick lateral shuffle to the other side, where they will pick up their partner's ball and throw it back. The return throw should be executed right from the floor with a full-body squat throw. Continue throwing for maximum distance and shuffling at maximum speed for 30 seconds. As your anaerobic conditioning improves, increase the drill time. The intensity of this excellent drill is rated 110 percent!

Full-Body Multi-Joint Medicine Ball Pass

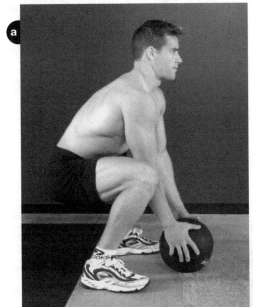

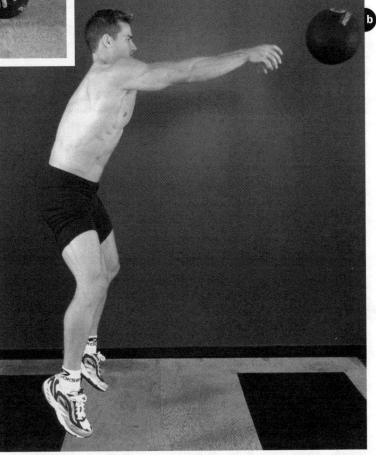

Medicine Ball Balance Catch

This exercise focuses on proprioception and balance during the eccentric loading and catch phase, as well as in the isometric post-catch position. It is a great way to integrate the entire body without having to handle an advanced load or advanced speed of movement.

Setup

Both partners stand on a balance board, facing each other, about two paces apart. Keep your feet shoulder-width apart, your knees slightly flexed, and your abdominals pre-contracted.

Movement

Send each other light passes, aimed at chest level and within the boundaries of each shoulder.

Finish

Receive the pass with a strong core and legs. Attempt to catch the ball while retaining your balance and remaining square to your partner. Be sure the knees stay in line over the ankles and do not drop in. Hold this balanced position for two seconds before returning each pass.

Advanced Progressions

Try these suggestions as you advance in this exercise. Use a full-body catch with static hold. Complete the same exercise setup. Upon catching the ball, progress into a full squat on the balance board. Hold the squat at the bottom position for three seconds before rising with a controlled motion to return the pass to your partner.

Catch passes outside the center of gravity. Complete the same exercise setup. Aim your light passes outside of your partner's center of gravity. Deliver passes outside of the shoulder boundary (off to the side), low passes, overhead passes, and short passes that fall in front of your partner. The catch-and-balance response is more challenging and is fun to try. Catch the ball and move back to a strong, well-balanced position before returning the pass.

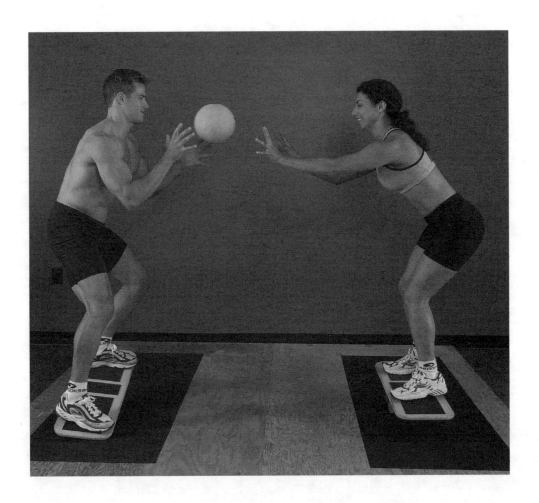

This is a great torso rotation exercise that also works the muscles eccentrically, building braking strength. The act of stopping and reversing direction helps to overload the torso musculature.

Setup

With a partner, stand back-to-back about six inches apart. Keep your feet shoulder-width apart, your knees slightly flexed, and your abdominals pre-contracted.

Movement

Holding the ball out away from his body, Partner A quickly rotates to his right *(a)*, then abruptly stops the ball and returns to the left, where he passes the ball to his partner *(b)*. Partner B picks up the ball on her right side and immediately rotates with speed to her left. Once the ball is on the left side, Partner B stops abruptly and quickly rotates back to the right side to drop off the ball.

Finish

Continue this sequence for a set number of repetitions. Repeat using the opposite hand to complete the pass.

Advanced Progression

Move your feet together, rather than shoulder-width apart. Keeping your knees bent, move the ball farther away from your body. Rotate and stop more quickly.

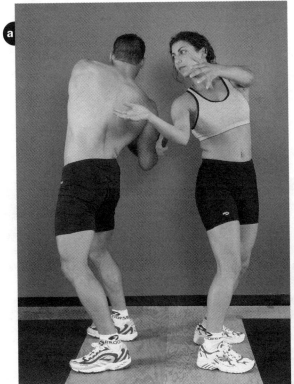

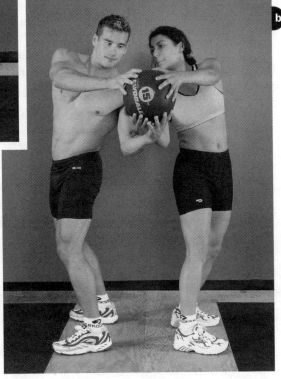

This exercise builds full-body power and torso rotation while producing sequential muscle firing for a smooth, multi-joint throw.

Setup

Stand with your back to your partner, about two paces apart. Keep your feet shoulder-width apart, your knees flexed, and your abdominals pre-contracted. Your partner is facing your back, one side step to the right.

Movement

Before you throw the ball, squat down and rotate until the ball is in front of your right shin. The throw is initiated from this position. Be sure to use a squat movement, dropping your hips to lower the ball to shin height, to avoid excessive forward trunk flexion. The throw begins at the foot, transfers through your right leg, moves through the hips and torso, and goes on to the upper body.

Remember, the desired ball direction is behind you to your partner, not just up, so you must rotate the torso and follow through. This will direct the ball from above your left shoulder to your partner, who is standing behind you and to your right *(a-b)*.

Finish

Your partner catches the ball and rolls it back to your right side. Pick it up and begin the sequential throw technique. Continue for the desired number of repetitions, then repeat the exercise, throwing over your right shoulder. Your partner will change his position, staying two paces behind you, but shifting to your left side.

Advanced Progression

After you release the throw, keep your hands up above your shoulders. Your partner will catch your throw and return a gentle pass into your hands. Complete the catch above your shoulders, rotate to the opposite side, squat, and then thrust upward to throw the ball back over the same shoulder.

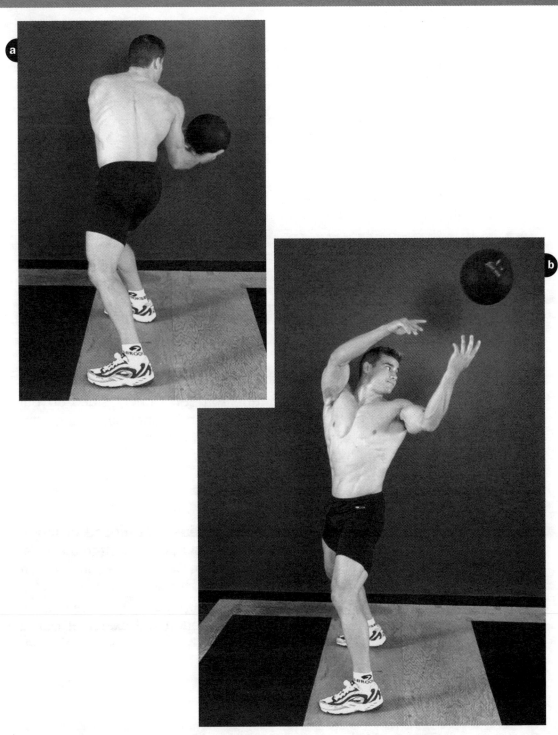

Left-to-right exercise produces excellent balance and proprioception responses, while overloading the speed center. The deep abdominal wall and core abdominal muscles contribute through eccentric loading, stabilization, and concentric action. The single-leg stance accelerates the demands on the speed center. You will feel every muscle working, from toes and ankles to legs, hips, and abdominals.

Setup

Stand on one leg, knee slightly flexed. Set the abdominals and focus on balance. Hold the ball with two hands in front of your body.

Movement

Move the ball to the left side of your body, but do not rotate the torso. The torso and shoulders should remain square, facing straight forward. Move the ball back across the body to the right side (a).

Finish

Continue to move the ball alternately from left to right sides of your body, reacting to the changing load position by contracting the abs, hips, and legs. Your degree of knee flexion will adjust accordingly to counterbalance the shifting load position.

Advanced Progressions

Try these strategies as you progress. Increase the speed of movement. Move the ball farther away from the body, farther off to the side, and farther in front of the body upon rotation. Or, toss the ball from left hand to right hand (b). Catch and absorb the throw with the arm, core, and leg. This increases the balance challenge as well as the loading on the abdominals. This is an excellent abdominal exercise! Use a rapid-fire toss. Move the ball from left to right as quickly as possible.

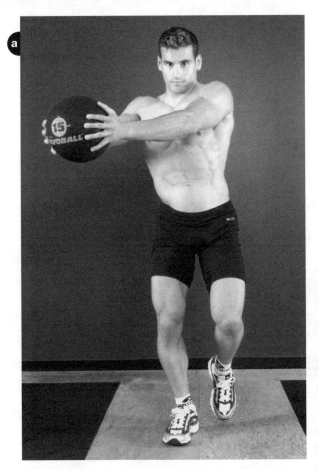

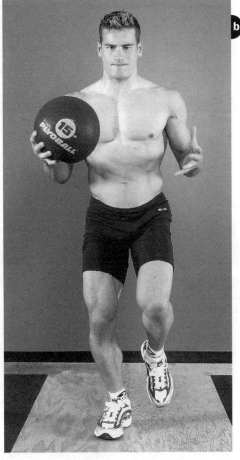

This power exercise loads the core and teaches sequential firing through the legs, hips, abdomen, and upper extremities.

Setup

Stand with feet at shoulder-width, facing your partner. Assume an athletic, ready position. Your partner holds a small medicine ball.

Movement

Your partner delivers a pass directly to one shoulder (a). As the ball approaches, step forward with one leg.

Finish

Upon making contact with the ball, immediately push the ball away from the body, straight out from your shoulder and back to your partner (b). Return to a ready position. Continue for a set number of repetitions. Upon making ball contact and initiating the push, remember, your hips and core—the speed center—must get behind this action and assist in force production.

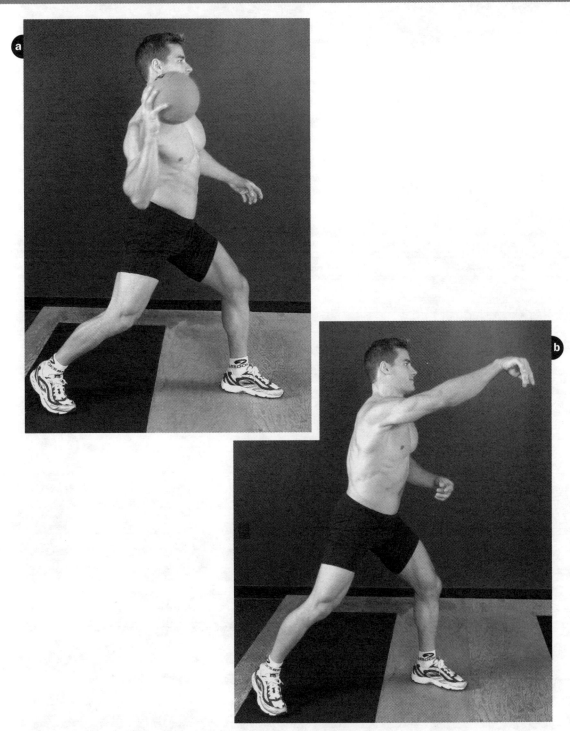

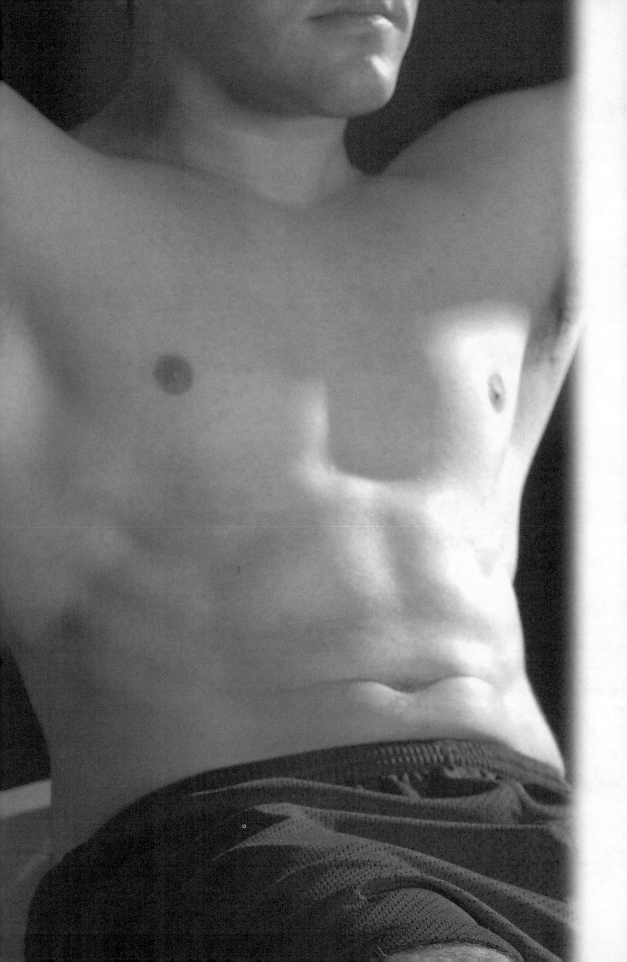

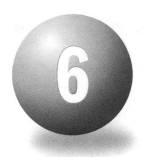

Abdominals and Lower Back

Performing crunches on a stability ball is one of the most effective abdominal exercises you will ever do. The shape of the ball pre-stretches the abdominals as you initiate the movement allowing the abdominals to work through a greater range of movement, resulting in more total work for these muscles. Crunches on the floor or on abdominal boards do not allow for this type of pre-stretch.

Setup

Sit atop the ball and slowly roll forward until your hips move off the ball. Continue rolling until your lower back is supported by the curve of the ball. Select a ball that will support your lower back, while allowing your head to extend back around the ball. Your hands should be beside your ears (a). Do not clasp your hands behind your head. If you have difficulty completing the crunch with your hands beside the ears, cross your arms over your chest.

Movement

After setting your abdominals, crunch forward until you are at approximately a 45-degree angle to the ball (b). It is important to maintain your neutral neck position, not allowing your chin to tuck down as you move.

Finish

Once you have reached the desired angle, slowly lower yourself back to the starting position. Continue for the desired number of repetitions.

Advanced Progressions

For a more advanced progression, add external weight to the exercise. This can be accomplished by holding a dumbbell on your chest or a cable behind your head. Once you have increased a chest weight to 25 or 30 pounds, however, you will need to anchor your feet to a solid object. This safety precaution will prevent you from rolling back over the ball with a weight load.

You can recruit more abdominal musculature by using a twist move during this exercise. From the starting position, as you crunch forward, focus on bringing your right elbow toward the left knee. Return to the starting position and repeat, bringing the left elbow toward the right knee.

Abdominal Crunch

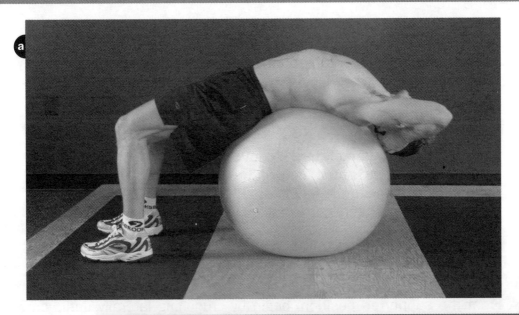

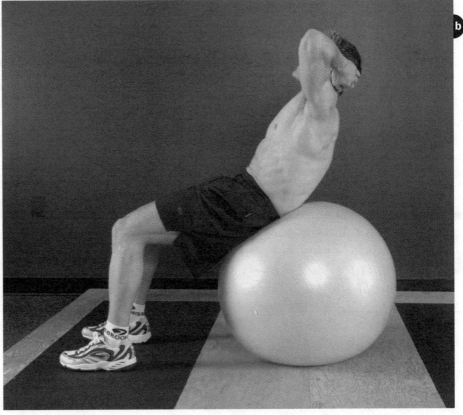

The abdominal side crunch focuses on the muscles that allow you to bend side to side, the oblique and quadratus lumborum musculature. These muscles are very important for the flexibility and stability of your core.

Setup

Place a ball approximately three to four feet from a wall. Sit on the ball so that your hips are at the apex of the ball, and your feet are against the wall. You will need the wall to stabilize your feet against so you do not roll forward. Lie across the ball so you are bending laterally over it *(a)*.

Movement

From the supported position, begin by crunching laterally until your knees, hips, and shoulders are all in line *(b)*.

Finish

Once your body is aligned, return to the starting position. Be sure to extend fully back over the ball.

Advanced Progression

As with the abdominal crunch, there are many variations of the side crunch. You can progress from completing the exercise with your arms across your chest, to placing your hands by your ears, to extending your arms over your head. You can also add external load by holding a dumbbell in front of your chest. By using a medicine ball to perform a side crunch throw to a partner, you can add a ballistic component to the drill *(c)*.

Abdominal Side Crunch

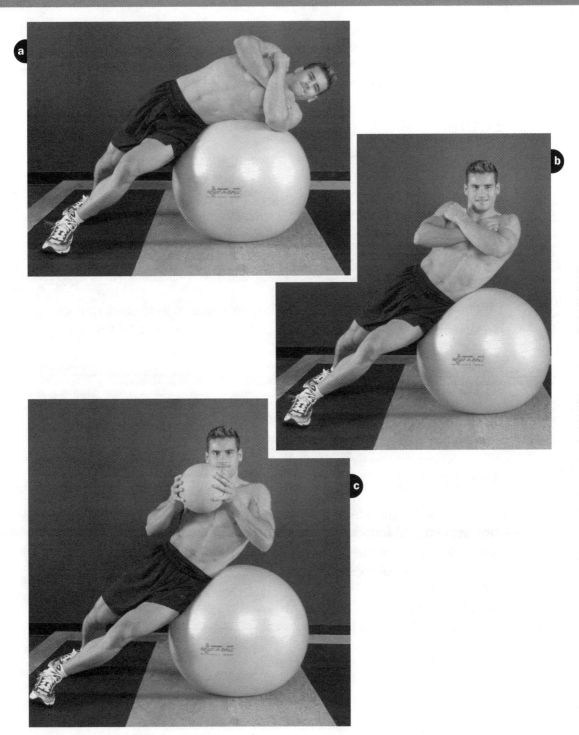

Supine Lower-Abdominal Cable Curl

The supine lower-abdominal cable curl is an effective method of using resistance to work the lower abdominal musculature. This area of the abdominals is important in controlling proper pelvic positioning, which can play a factor in decreasing lower back pain.

Setup

Lying on the floor with your legs over the ball, place a cable with an ankle strap around your ankles. Your hands should be under your lower back at the navel level. Make sure that your back maintains contact with your hands to ensure proper lower back posture during this exercise.

Movement

Begin by setting your core, and bring your knees in toward your chest. Focus on not allowing your back to arch off the ground as you bring your knees up and back.

Finish

Continue to flex at the knee until your legs are slightly past a 90-degree angle. Then, slowly return to the start position.

Safety Note

If you cannot maintain your posture with the added load of the cable, then you should focus on performing the movement without the cable. Once you can execute this successfully, progress to using a medicine ball between your legs, and then try again to perform the movement with the cable.

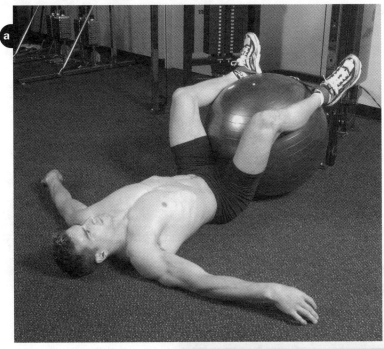

Supine Lower-Abdominal Curl and Crunch

The supine lower-abdominal curl and crunch is the most advanced lower-abdominal exercise you will perform. It focuses on pelvic strength, stability, and balance.

Setup

To begin, set a ball in front of something solid you can hold onto. The side of a power rack or a loaded barbell will do. Lie over the ball with your knees bent and your lower back supported by the curve of the ball. Hold on to a rack overhead to stabilize yourself (a).

Movement

To initiate movement, begin by setting your core, and focus on uncurling your pelvis off the curve of the ball. You will accomplish this by slowly bringing your knees toward you (b). As your legs reach a 90-degree angle, you will then attempt to touch the ceiling with your knees by lifting your pelvis higher in a reverse crunch position (c).

Finish

Once you have reached as high as possible, hold your position for two to three seconds, and then slowly return to the beginning position by reversing your movements.

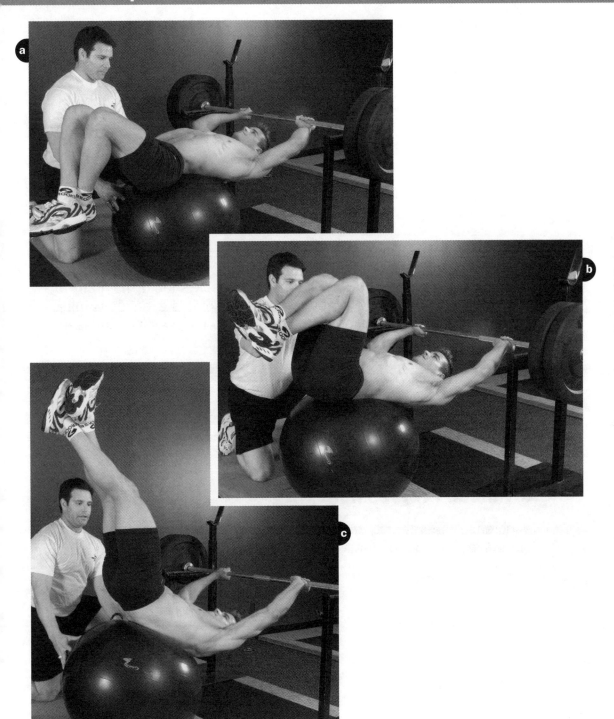

The reverse back extension focuses on the posterior chain muscles, which include the hamstrings, gluteals, and lower-back erectors. These muscles allow the back and legs to function as a unit. The regular back extension should be used if you are not strong enough to extend your hips up and back. The back extension uses the stability ball in the same motions as described here.

Setup

Place a Swiss ball on top of the Sorinex bench. Lie over the ball in a prone position, grasping the front handles for support (a).

Movement

Begin by setting your core. Your head and neck should maintain a neutral position. To ensure that the movement of this exercise is initiated by your glutes, it is important to activate them with a squeeze before beginning to extend your hips and legs (b).

Finish

The legs should be raised until the knees, hips, and shoulders are aligned. Hold the contracted position for a second, then lower to the original position.

Advanced Progression

To increase the intensity of this exercise, place a dumbbell between your ankles for added load.

Sorinex Reverse Back Extension

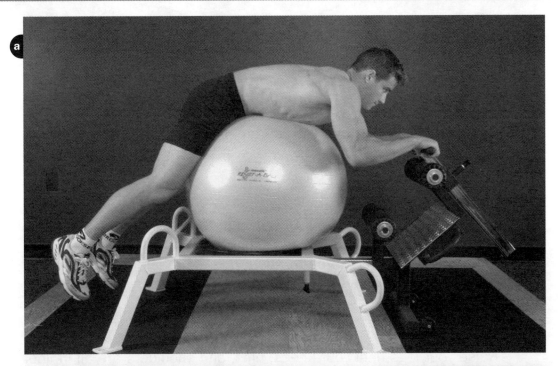

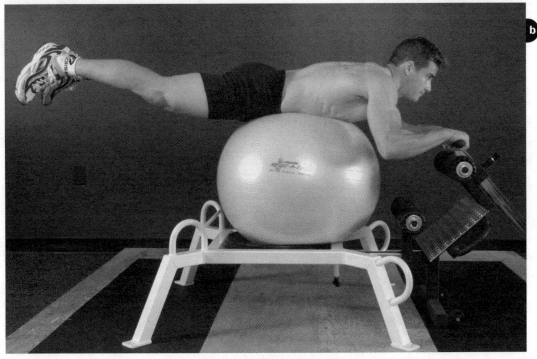

If you do not have access to the Sorinex stability ball bench, you can still perform the reverse back extension using a flat bench.

Setup

Place a Swiss ball on top of a flat bench. Connect an adjustable cable to your ankles and lie over the ball, grasping the sides of the bench for support.

Movement

Begin by setting your core. As with the Sorinex reverse back extension, your head and neck should maintain a neutral position, and you should activate your glutes by squeezing them before beginning the hip and leg extension movement *(a)*.

Finish

Raise your legs until your knees, hips, and shoulders are all in line. Hold the contracted position for a second, then lower to the original position *(b)*.

Advanced Progressions

The reverse extension can be slowly attained as the end of a long, safe progression. The following are some examples:

1. Begin with a ball on the floor. Brace your hands on the floor for balance, then extend your hips. Begin with an under-inflated ball and progress to full inflation.
2. Place the ball on a bench and perform movement with no external resistance. Again, begin with an under-inflated ball and progress to full inflation.
3. As in the previous tip, hold a 5- to 10-pound dumbbell between the ankles and extend the hips. This is the same as number 2 but you are adding a 5- to 10-pound load.
4. Progress to performing a full reverse hyperextension using a cable, as described in the preceding drill.

Reverse Back Extension

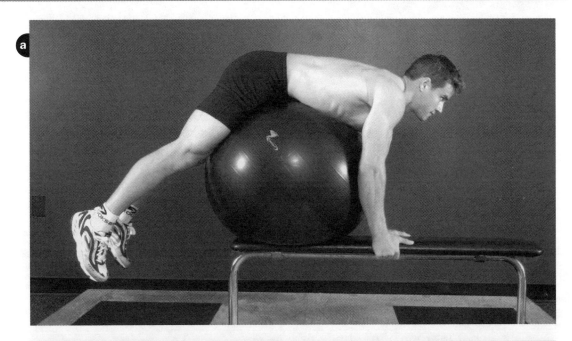

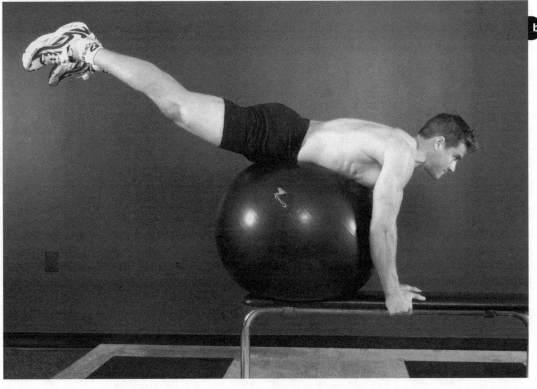

This is a good warm-up exercise, since it gently works the legs, hips, torso, and upper body. With more powerful passes, it is a great torso rotation strength exercise, pertinent to many sports.

Setup

Partners stand four strides apart, both facing the same wall. One partner has a medicine ball. Feet are positioned shoulder-width apart, while the knees are flexed, and abdominals are set. The partners should turn their heads to see each other.

Movement

All parts of the body work together to produce the rotation pass. Push off your outside foot and transfer the force through the hips and into torso rotation, while the arms draw the ball across your body. Release the ball with a full follow-through, aiming the ball so your partner can catch it in front of her body *(a)*.

Finish

Catch the ball with a strong core to protect the lower back. Absorb the catch by flexing the knee of the outside leg, rotating the torso to the outside, and allowing the arms to travel across the body to an exaggerated position at the side *(b)*. Stop and reverse the process to return the pass to your partner.

Advanced Progression

Receive the ball with a static catch. Flex the knees a little more to prepare to catch the ball in front of your body, and use the abdominals to completely brake the path of the ball. Catch the ball, stopping its travel right in front of your body. Once stationary, move back into the normal catch reception position to prepare to throw the ball back to your partner.

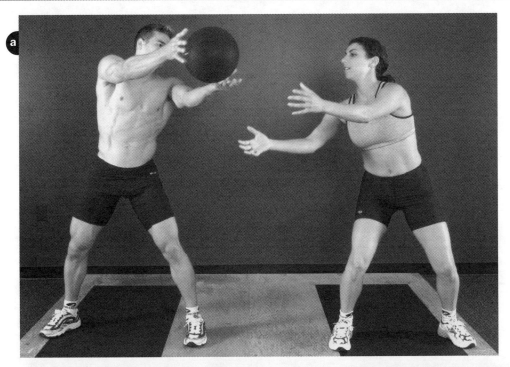

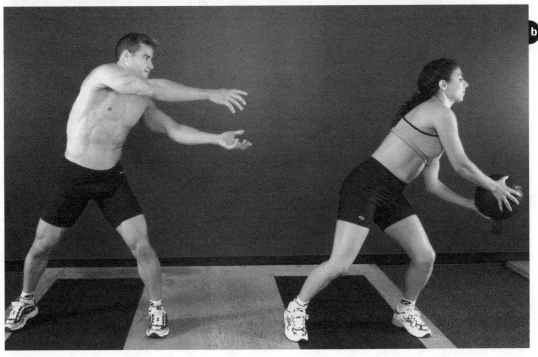

This is simply a good abdominal exercise that prepares the torso for more dynamic rotation exercises and more intense eccentric loading.

Setup

Sit on the ground, leaning back one third of the way into a sit-up. Your feet should remain on the ground with your knees flexed. Hold a medicine ball in front of your body.

Movement

Rotate to the left as far as comfortably possible. Touch the ball to the ground out and away from your body *(a)*.

Finish

Lift the ball back off the ground and rotate around to the right, carrying the ball across the body. Touch it to the ground on your right *(b)*.

Advanced Progressions

The farther away from the body the ball is carried and touched to the floor, the greater the load on the abdominal muscles. An intense progression involves lifting the feet off the ground. Maintain knee flexion to 90 degrees, hold the legs and feet together, and complete the same exercise while holding the feet a few inches in the air. You will need a stronger core both to lift the ball back off the ground and to stabilize the body and hold position while rotating.

V-Sit and Rotate

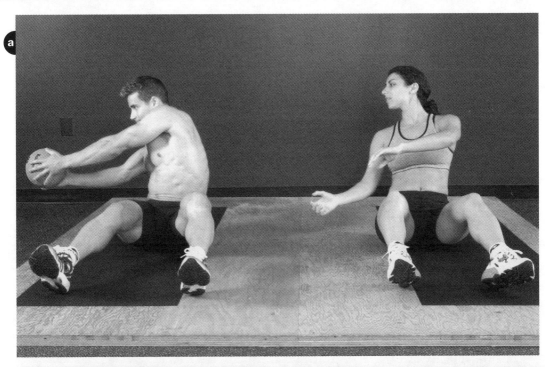

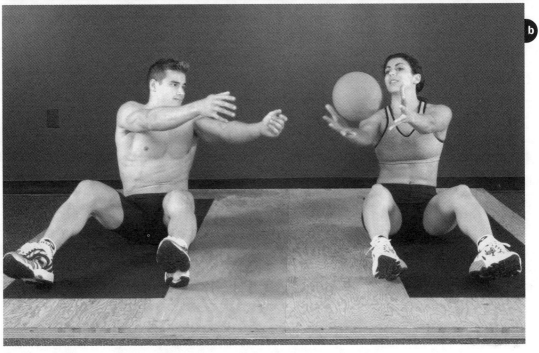

Standing torso rotation is a vital movement pattern to overload and strengthen the muscles in preparation for sport actions as well as real life activity.

Setup

With a partner, stand back to back, about six inches apart. Keep your feet shoulder-width apart, your knees slightly flexed, and your abdominals pre-contracted.

Movement

Partner A rotates to his right and passes the ball to Partner B, who receives it on her left side *(a)*. Partner B receives the ball and holds it out away from her torso. Partner B then rotates to the right and returns the pass to Partner A, who receives it on his left *(b)*. A key to this exercise is maintaining a strong core and bent knees so that the rotation comes from the hips and abdomen. You should feel your core leading the way.

Finish

Continue this sequence for a set number of repetitions. Repeat the exercise, passing in the opposite direction.

Advanced Progression

Rotate a full 360 degrees. The partners should move about two feet apart and remain back to back. The extra distance leaves room for the ball and for hip movement, as the pass will now transfer behind the back between partners. Partner A rotates to the right and continues twisting to position the ball behind his back. Partner B rotates to the opposite side, turning to her right to pick up the pass behind her back. Partner B next rotates to the left, holding the ball out away from her body. After dropping off the ball, Partner A also rotates to his left to be in position to receive the return pass.

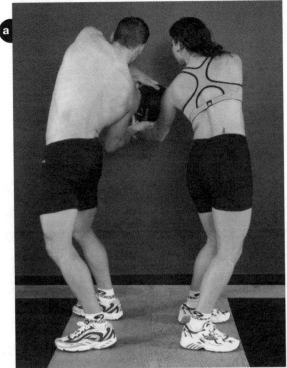

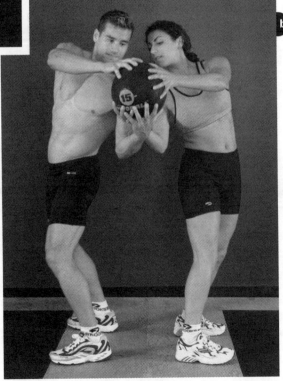

Sorinex Russian Twist

The Russian twist, performed on the Sorinex bench, can provide the greatest challenge to the twisting and stabilizing muscles of the core in terms of both strength and power.

Setup

Place the ball on top of the Sorinex bench, and hook your ankles under the ankle supports. Your glutes and hamstrings should be on top of the ball. You will be slightly flexed at the hips *(a)*.

Movement

Begin by setting your abdominals. Then rotate all the way to one side *(b)*. An attempt should be made to ensure that rotation is initiated by the core. It is also very important to focus your eyes on your hands, enhancing the total core rotation as you move.

Finish

As you reach the end of your range, you will begin moving in the opposite direction. This movement should be executed quickly, which will enhance the power component of this exercise.

Advanced Progressions

Add a medicine ball or a dumbbell to the hands. Using a medicine ball, ballistically rotate to one side and throw the ball to a partner. The partner will throw the ball back when your hands are in position over your chest. At this point you will take the ball back into rotation, decelerate, and release again.

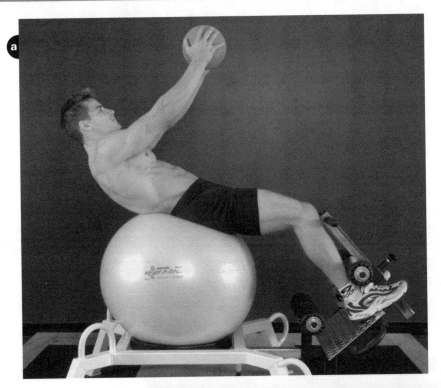

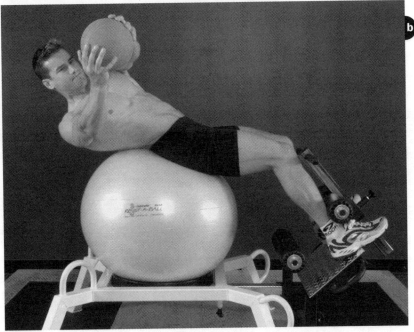

The Russian twist is an excellent exercise for integrating static extension and rotational trunk movement. Movement of this nature occurs in many sports, including football, rugby, hockey, and tennis.

Setup

Sitting on a ball, walk forward, allowing the ball to roll underneath you. Keep walking out until your head and shoulders are supported by the ball. Your arms should be extended over your chest, your abdominals set, and your core parallel to the ground *(a)*.

Movement

Begin by rotating all the way to one side *(b-c)*. An attempt should be made to ensure that rotation is initiated by the core. Many first-timers to the twist will initiate rotation from the shoulder. As mentioned for the Sorinex Russian twist, it is also very important to keep your eyes on your hands, enhancing the total core rotation as you move.

Finish

As you reach the end of your range, begin moving in the opposite direction.

Advanced Progressions

Hold a medicine ball or dumbbell in your hand. Set up in front of an adjustable cable. The constant loading from the cable will allow you to obtain greater loading in both directions.

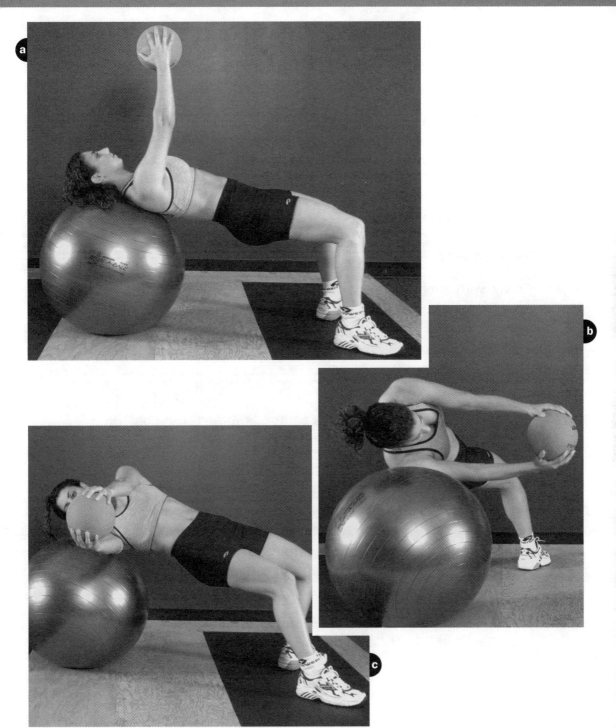

This exercise places a weight at the end of a lever arm to increase demand on the torso to stabilize and direct movement.

Setup

Lie on the floor in a supine position, with your arms straight out to the sides. Make sure you achieve a solid pelvic tilt. Set the abdominals before lifting the legs into the air. Legs should be held together and flexed to 90 degrees. Place a small medicine ball between your knees. Press inward to hold the ball in place and to activate your adductor and hip musculature (a).

Movement

Slowly, with a controlled movement, lower the knees off to the left side. Shoulders and back must remain flat on the floor (b).

Finish

Lift the legs, still flexed, back up over your hips and to the right side. Lower to the right. Stop and return. Continue for the desired number of repetitions or until you lose a neutral, supine torso position.

Advanced Progressions

Complete the same sequence with more speed. Drop legs to the left, and activate muscles to decelerate and stop before touching the ground. Return across the body to the opposite side.

Position the legs straight over the body and the ball between the ankles (c). This will increase the lever arm and place the loading farther out on the lever.

The Twister

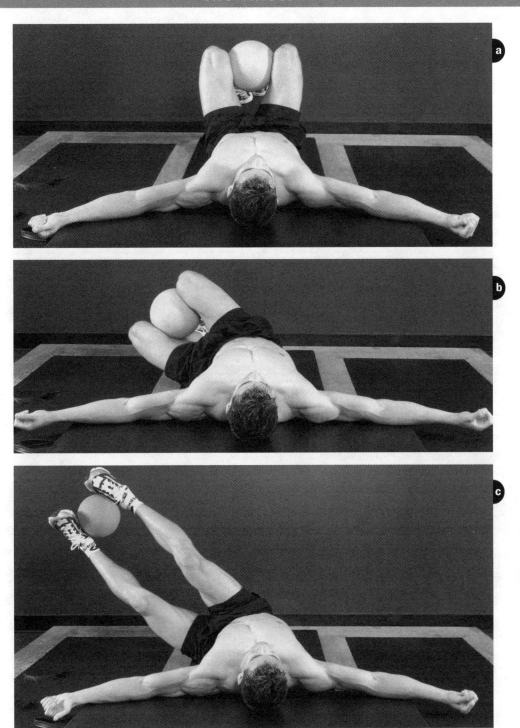

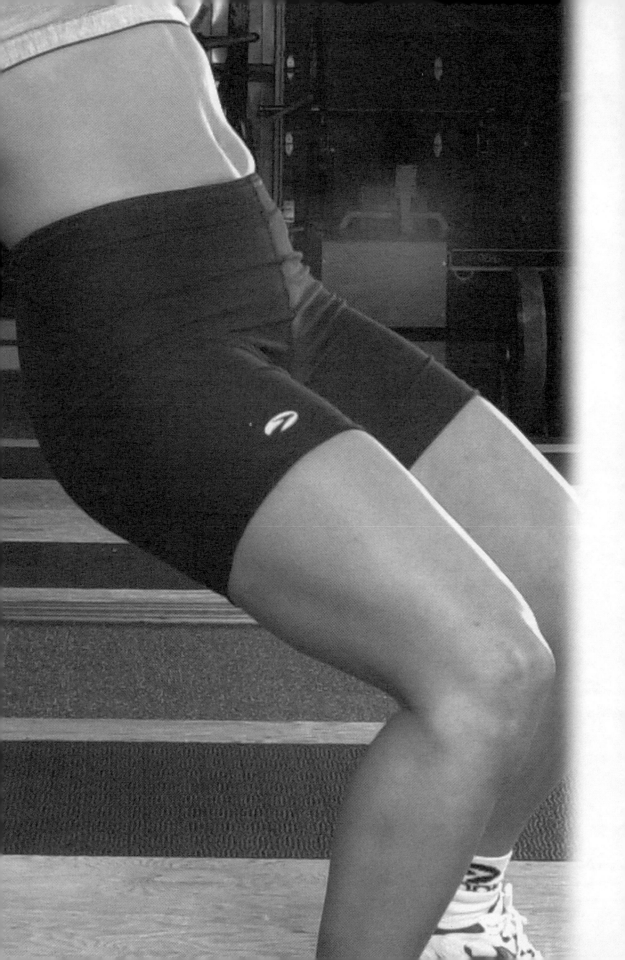

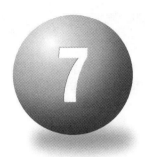

Legs
and Hips

The hip extension knee flexion is an exercise that can work your hamstrings as both a knee flexor and hip extensor, making it extremely productive.

Setup

Lying supine on the ground, place a ball under your heels. Place your arms in a T position to assist with balance *(a)*.

Movement

Movement is initiated by squeezing your glutes and raising your hips off the ground *(b)*. Once your ankles, knees, and hips are aligned, bring your heels toward you by flexing at the knee *(c)*.

Finish

Once your heels are at the end of their range, reverse the movement. After extending your knees, lower your hips.

Advanced Progressions

Move your arms in to your side to increase the challenge of balance. By using a larger ball, you will increase your range of motion as well as the balance challenge.

Add a cable or surgical tubing around your ankles to increase the load as your knees flex.

Try using a single-leg movement instead of double-leg movement.

Hip Extension Knee Flexion

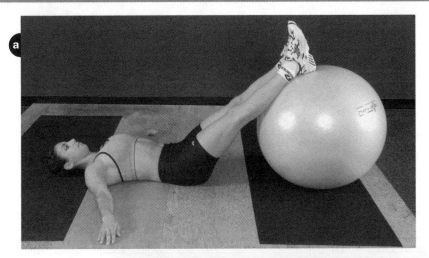

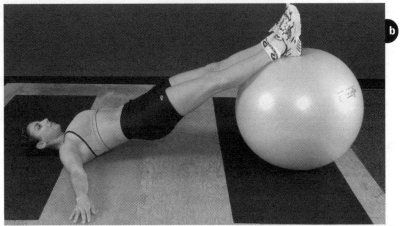

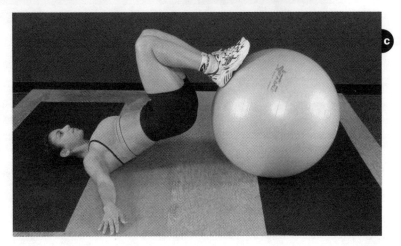

The supine leg cable curl is another great method of working the hamstring from both the hip and the knee.

Setup

Place the ball under your shoulders. Hold on to a cable or surgical tubing placed behind your head *(a)*. You will need to ensure that your heels are on a non-slip surface, or are placed in front of something solid like a weight bar.

Movement

The movement begins by bringing up the hips until the body is parallel to the ground. Once you are in this position, you will flex at your knees, rolling forward on the ball *(b)*.

Finish

Roll as far forward as possible, maintaining good posture and form. Reverse the movement by extending the knees. As you come back to full knee extension, do not drop your hips, but prepare to go into the next repetition.

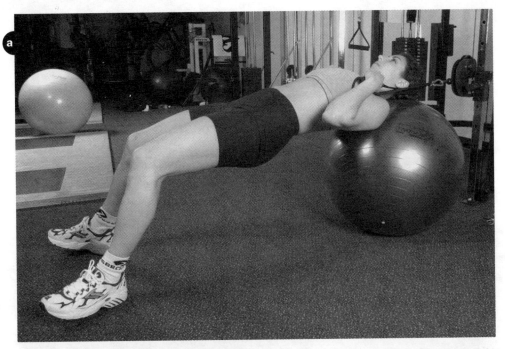

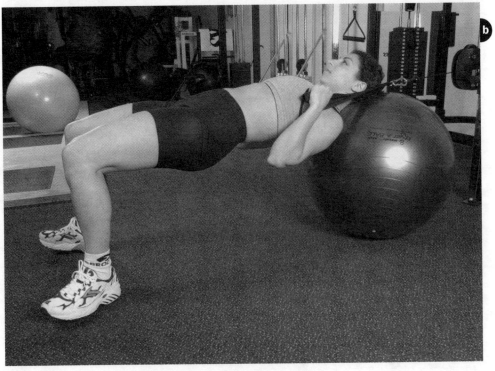

The split squat is a great overall exercise for the muscles in the legs and hips. It also requires the postural muscles to fire, keeping the torso upright and square.

Setup

Stand in front of a ball and place the back of the right foot atop the ball. Shuffle your left foot forward and shift your weight onto this support leg. The front supporting foot points forward, so your knee will track straight over the ankle. Contract your core to help hold a strong balance position *(a)*.

Movement

Drop your hips and roll your right leg back until the support leg is flexed to 90 degrees. Hold this position for two seconds. Make sure the knee of your support leg is not past your toes—if it is, your stance is too short. To correct this, shuffle your support foot farther forward *(b)*.

Finish

Using the muscles in your support leg, extend the leg to elevate your body back to the setup position. Stay strong and centered to avoid any torso sway as you come back up. Complete the set, switch legs, and repeat.

Spotting Tips

Beginners will need a light spot for this exercise. The spotter should place his hands on each side of the ball to provide stability.

Advanced Progression

Place the front support foot on a balance board to create dual instability *(c)*.

Split Squat

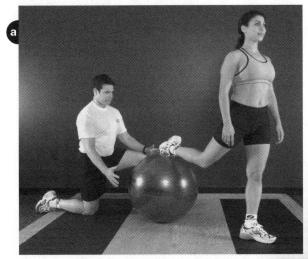

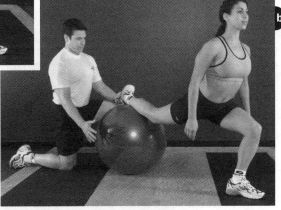

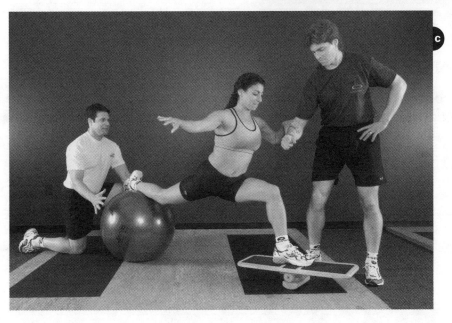

The wall squat unloads some of your body weight, which helps athletes prepare to progress to free-weight squats. You will activate all of the major leg muscles with this exercise.

Setup

Stand facing away from a wall. Place a stability ball against the wall at low back height. Plant your feet 12 inches in front of your body with a shoulder-width stance, toes pointing forward *(a)*. This exercise can be used with or without dumbbells.

Movement

Leaning into the ball, lower your body until your knees are flexed at a 90-degree angle. Hold this position for two seconds. As you squat, the ball will move to your mid- and upper-back region. Note your feet—your weight should be on your heels, not your toes, and your knees should not be out past your toes. Except to check your knee position, keep your head and eyes up *(b)*.

Finish

Extend your legs to elevate your body back to the setup position.

Advanced Progression

At the bottom of the squat, lift one foot off the ground and hold for five seconds *(c)*. Switch feet and repeat this motion. Maintain your balance and hip position with one-foot support.

Wall Squat

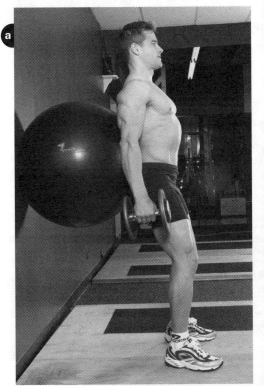

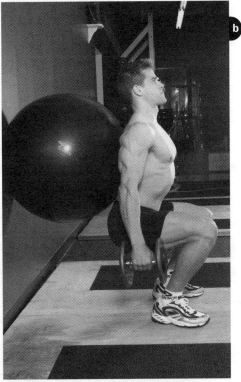

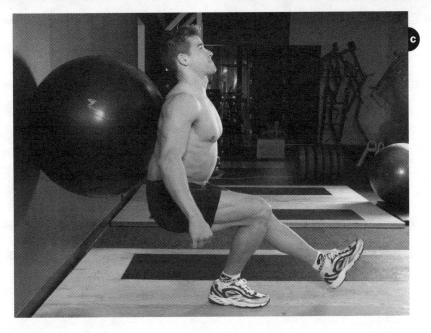

The lateral wall squat functions to build more sport-specific strength. It replicates the angles needed for lateral movement and stopping. The glutes, hamstrings, and quadriceps are the main beneficiaries.

Setup

Stand sideways beside a wall. Position a stability ball against the wall at elbow height. Lean against the ball at a 45-degree angle, with your outside leg supporting your body weight *(a)*.

Movement

Lower into a one-leg squat position, maintaining the 45-degree angle and leaning into the ball. As you flex your knee and lower your hips, the ball will move from elbow height to shoulder height. Keep your hips and shoulders as square as possible *(b)*. Rotate the opposite direction and repeat with both legs. Repeat the exercise using your inside leg.

Finish

Using the muscles in your support leg, extend the leg to elevate your body back to the setup position.

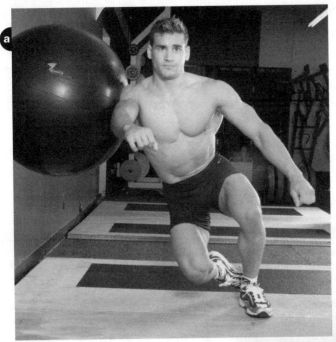

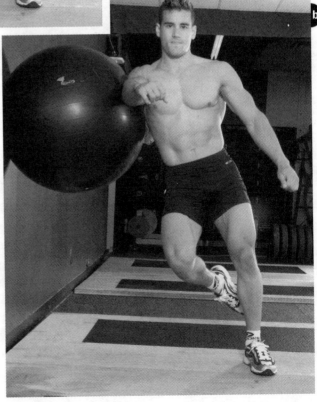

The inner and outer thigh are areas that athletes have always had difficulty training. Most exercises for these areas are completed with the foot off the ground, as in the use of a multi-hip machine or cable attachments. However, these muscles are used in movement, while the foot is in contact with the ground. The leg blaster can avoid this problem by training the muscles in the appropriate manner.

Setup

You will need to set up close to an adjustable cable column, using a 45-centimeter ball. With your foot sitting atop the ball, place a cable belt around your inside ankle. The outside leg will be planted, and should maintain a bent-knee position. Your hips should be back and your abdominals set. This setup method will emphasize the inner thigh and quads *(a)*.

Movement

The initial movement that activates the inner thigh muscles comes from the inside of the foot pressing down on the ball. Once you have established this pressure, roll the ball toward you by bringing in your hip *(b)*. It is very important that you keep your hips back and maintain a natural curve in your lower back. Other movements include figure 8s and circles.

Finish

Return to the starting position by releasing your leg, allowing a full range of movement on the return.

Alternate Method

You can focus on the outer, rather than inner, thigh muscles by placing the cable on the opposite leg described previously. The movement and sequence for the exercise is the same. The main difference is that you will be pushing out rather than pulling in.

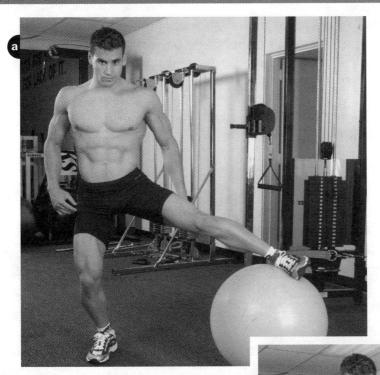

Lunge With Medicine Ball Pass

This excellent, complex exercise takes an important leg-strength drill and adds an element to increase upper-body power.

Setup

Partners face each other, about three or four strides apart. One partner has a medicine ball *(a)*.

Movement

Holding the ball, lift one leg off the ground. While flexing at the hip and knee, cycle the leg forward and softly plant it on the ground in front of the body. The lunge length should be long enough to produce a 90-degree angle at the knee. The knee should not be positioned out past your toes. Lower your leg until your thigh is parallel to the ground. Before planting your foot, pass the ball to your partner *(b)*.

Finish

Hold the lunge position and focus on remaining well balanced. While receiving the return pass, push off with your lead foot to return to the starting position.

Advanced Progression

Progress to using a lunge and catch. One partner lunges and catches while the other throws. Lunge alternately with the left and right leg, while receiving passes at random. Your partner passes from directly in front of you to a variety of places outside your midline, and also moves her position off to the side to deliver passes across your body. Catch, balance, and hold for two seconds before returning the ball to your partner and taking your next lunge step.

Lunge With Medicine Ball Pass

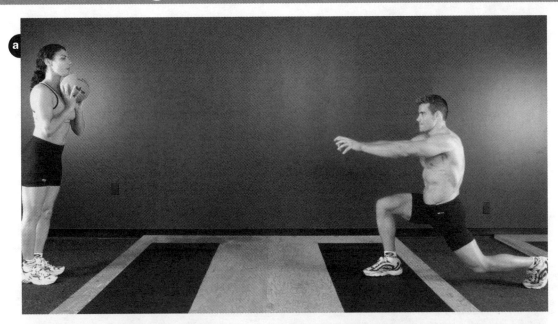

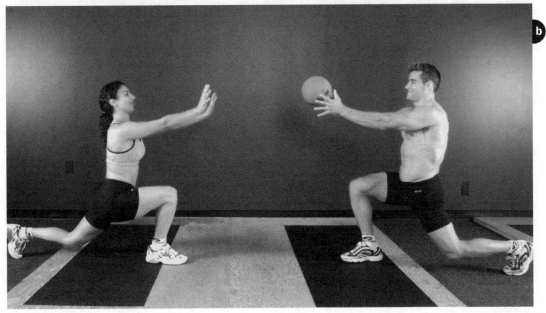

This exercise builds strength and dynamic flexibility in the legs, hips, and torso, linking these muscles together.

Setup

Stand upright, holding the ball just below chest height.

Movement

Lift your right leg, flexing at the hip and knee, and cycle it forward to softly plant it on the ground in front of the body *(a)*. The lunge length should produce a 90-degree angle at the knee without allowing your knee to be positioned out past your toes. Your thigh should be parallel to the ground. As you land, shift your weight to the right.

Finish

Push off with the left foot to return to an upright position, and continue forward with the left leg into a lunge. As you land, rotate your weight over to the left *(b)*. Continue for the set number of repetitions.

Advanced Progression

Lunge and rotate with arms extended. Hold the ball as far away from your torso as possible. The farther away the ball is held from your torso and center of gravity, the longer the lever arm, thereby placing greater load on your shoulders, back, and torso.

Walking Lunge and Rotate

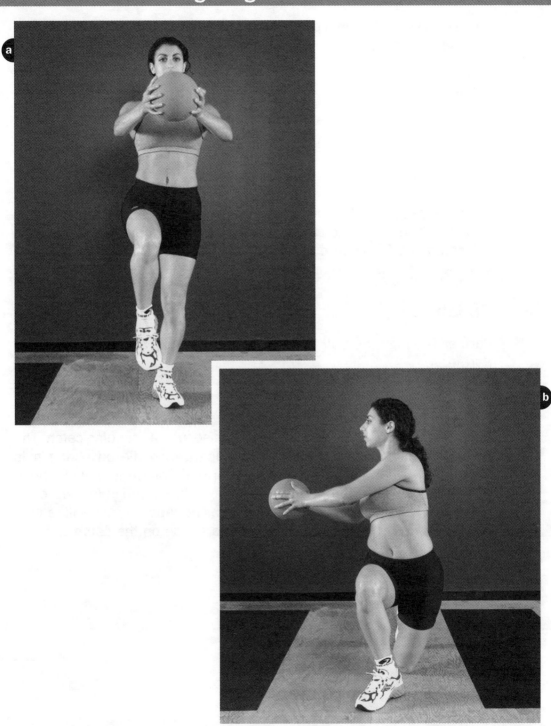

This exercise works the hips and torso with frontal-plane loading through side flexion of the trunk.

Setup

Partners stand four feet apart, both facing the same wall. One partner has a medicine ball. They begin in an upright kneeling position.

Movement

Partner A passes to Partner B *(a)*. Partner B catches the ball above his head and about one inch in front of his body. Partner B should absorb the catch and follow through as far as possible to the opposite side, while keeping his torso upright *(b)*.

Finish

Partner B brings the ball back over her head and returns the pass to Partner A.

Advanced Progression

Rather than kneeling to perform the exercise, use a standing catch. The feet should be positioned shoulder-width apart, knees flexed, abdominals set, and the head turned to see your partner. Catch the ball overhead and about one inch in front of the body, but follow through farther to the opposite side. If accuracy allows, move farther apart, which will require more power for the throw and provide more load on the catch.

Kneeling Side Pass

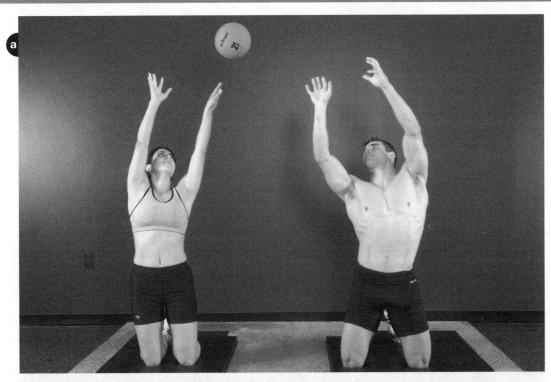

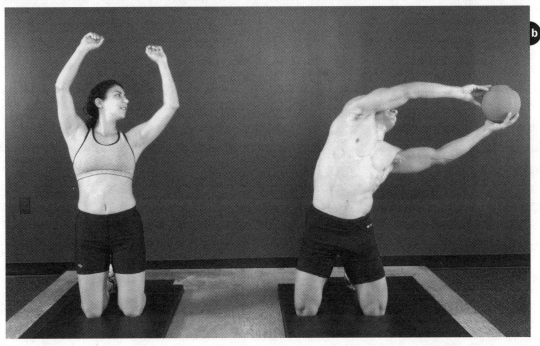

You will feel the benefit of this great, full-body exercise in the legs, back, core, and shoulders.

Setup

Stand with feet shoulder-width apart, holding a medicine ball in front of your body with both hands.

Movement

Step out to the left and lower into a lateral squat position, shifting your body weight over your left leg. As you lower your body to the left, push the medicine ball away from your chest until your arms are fully extended. Hold this position for two seconds.

Finish

Push off with the left leg to move back into a neutral stance. As you push off, pull the ball back toward your chest. Next, step out to the right and lower into a side squat position, extending your arms to push the ball away from your chest as before. Hold the position for two seconds. Push off with the right leg and pull the ball in to return to the start position.

Advanced Progression

You can progress with ball weights.

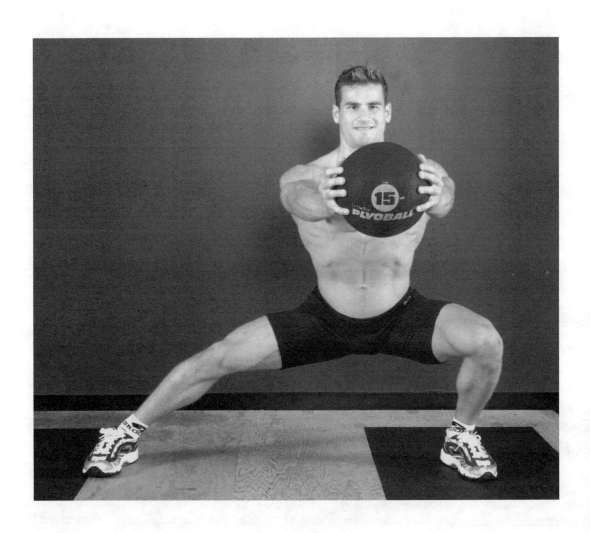

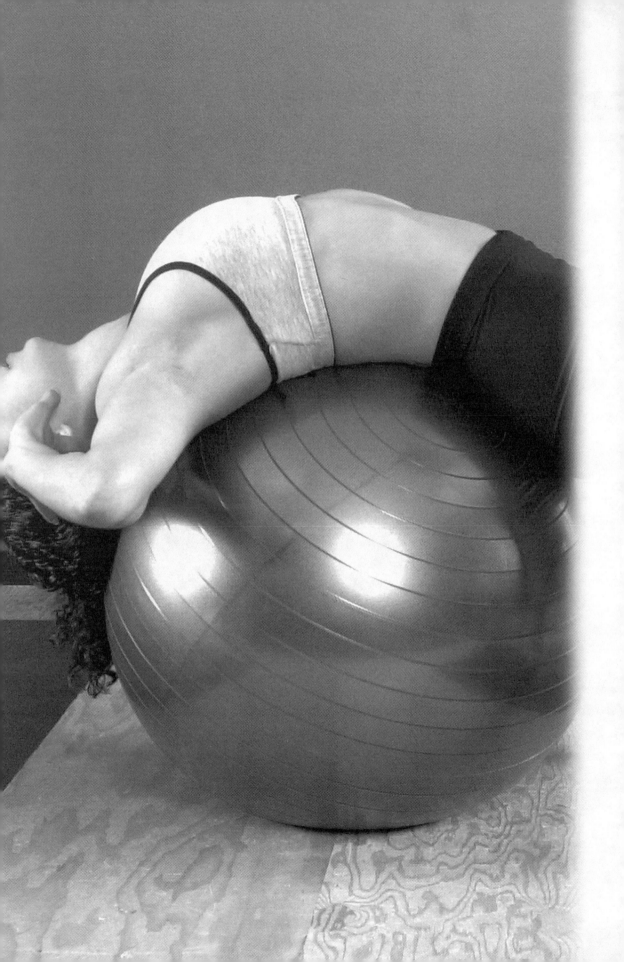

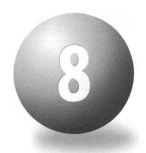

Flexibility Exercises

Mobility in the spine is essential if the rest of the body is to function efficiently. As in strengthening, stretching the spine from multiple planes and angles will assist in spinal health. The spinal extension provides a safe method for stretching the anterior ligaments and muscles of the spinal column as well as the abdominal muscles.

Setup

Sitting on a ball, walk forward until the natural curve of your lower back is over the ball *(a)*.

Movement

Begin to rock back and forth by pressing your legs into the floor. This will force the ball to roll back *(b)*. Following the roll of the ball will stretch the abdominal muscles. The farther back you roll, the greater the stretch. Begin with smaller rolls, then progress to larger ones.

Finish

Once you have reached the end of your range, hold the stretch for 8 to 15 seconds, and then return to your original position. This hold time is shorter than in most stretches, because the position of the head may cause dizziness if the stretch is maintained for an extended period of time.

Spinal Extension

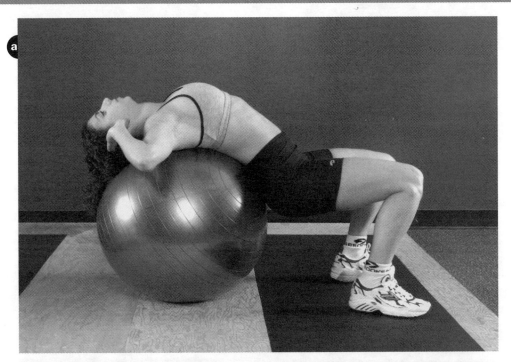

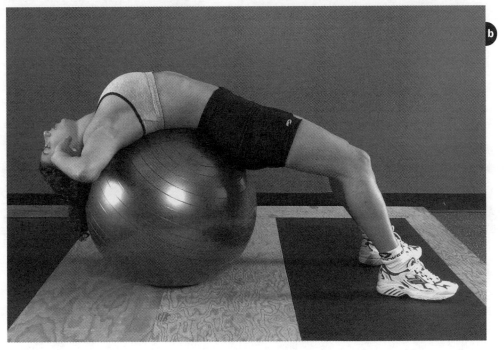

This drill will stretch the side-flexing spinal muscles along with the obliques.

Setup

Place a ball approximately three to four feet from a wall. Sit on the ball so that your hips are atop the ball and your feet are against the wall. You will need the wall to stabilize your feet so that you do not roll forward. Lie in a lateral position over the ball.

Movement

There is no movement once you have reached the stretched position.

Finish

Hold the stretched position over the ball for 20 to 30 seconds, then repeat the exercise on the opposite side.

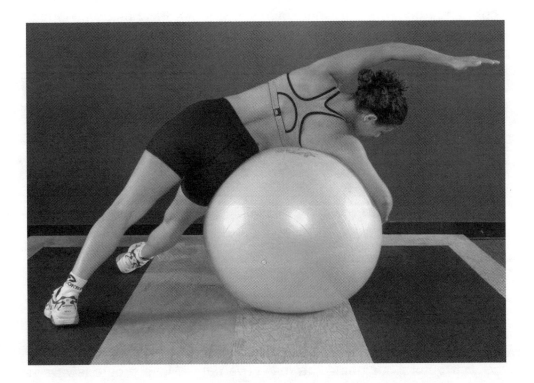

Supine Hamstring Stretch

The hamstrings, which are found on the back of the thigh, are typically some of the tightest muscles in the body, limiting flexibility around the hip and lower back. The supine hamstring stretch will provide a static and a dynamic challenge for the hamstring muscle group at both the hip and knee joint.

Setup

With your knees bent, place a ball between your feet and the wall. If your hamstrings are very inflexible, you will need to position yourself farther back from the wall *(a)*.

Movement

Keeping your pelvis in contact with the floor, begin to roll the ball up the wall by extending your legs *(b)*. Once your legs are fully extended, hold your position for 20 to 30 seconds and then return to the start position. You can also perform dynamic stretches by moving the ball more quickly in an up and down motion.

Finish

Perform 15 to 20 movements before resting. Flex at the knees, drawing the heels back towards the floor.

Advanced Progression

As you become more flexible, you will want to slide your body closer to the wall before beginning the leg movement. Move progressively in small increments to prevent your pelvis from coming off the floor as you move closer.

Supine Hamstring Stretch

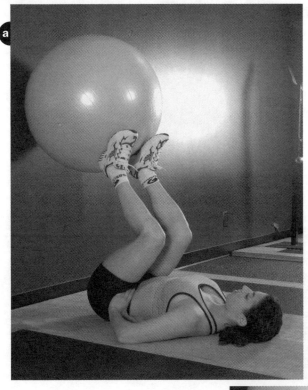

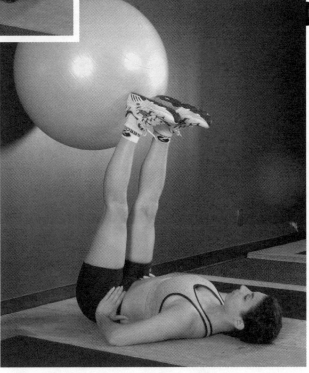

Stretching the hamstring from a standing position will provide more emphasis to the part of the muscle closer to the hip.

Setup

Place your foot on top of a ball.

Movement

Maintain the lordotic curve in your lower back and slowly flex forward. Focus on moving your navel toward your thigh. As you flex forward, press your heel into the ball with approximately 30-percent pressure. Hold this contraction for five to six seconds, relax the stretch for two seconds, and then proceed to the next stretch. This system utilizes the PNF method of stretching, which basically implies that if you contract a muscle, allow it to relax, and then stretch it again, the subsequent stretch will be greater. You can also focus on the different heads of the hamstring by pointing your toes in or out.

Finish

Perform three to five static stretches of 20 to 30 seconds each, or two to three sets of three to four PNF stretches each.

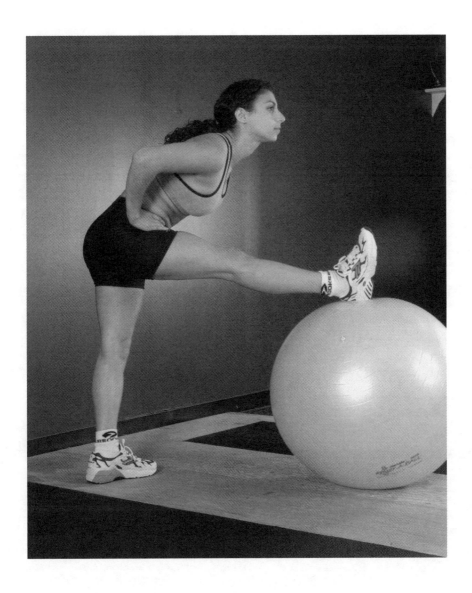

The latissimus dorsi and pectorals are two muscle groups that, if not stretched efficiently, can restrict range of motion in the shoulder. Flexibility in these areas is key for any throwing athlete and for overall shoulder health.

Setup

Take a split stance with your right foot forward and place a ball between your left hand and the wall *(a)*.

Movement

Begin by rolling the ball straight up the wall until your arm is fully extended *(b)*. To increase the stretch on your shoulder, lunge forward slightly. Hold the stretch for 20 to 30 seconds and then return to your original position. You can also perform this dynamically by increasing the speed of the ball roll and lunge.

Finish

Perform three to five static stretches of 20 to 30 seconds each, or two to three sets of 10 dynamic stretches each.

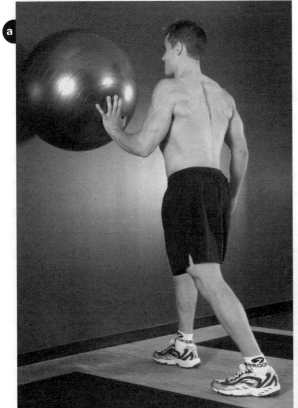

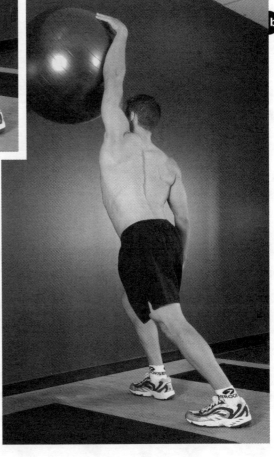

Stretching the posterior side of the shoulder is important for mobility and range of shoulder movement.

Setup

Kneel in front of a ball, with the ball slightly off to your left. Reach across your body to place your right hand on the ball *(a)*.

Movement

Begin to roll the ball to the left by pushing with the right hand. As you reach the end of your range, flex forward *(b)*. This will place greater stretch on the posterior fibers of the deltoid and the rhomboid, which span the space between your shoulder blade and your upper spine.

Finish

Hold the stretch for 20 to 30 seconds and then return to your initial position. Repeat three to five times.

Kneeling Posterior Shoulder Stretch

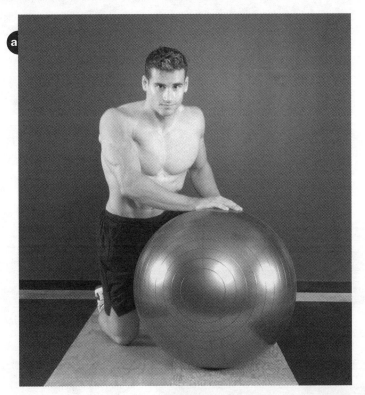

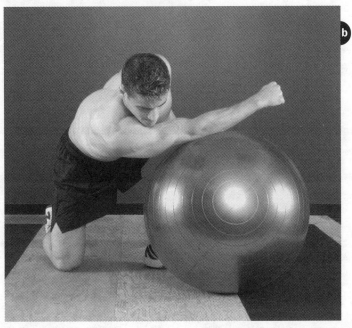

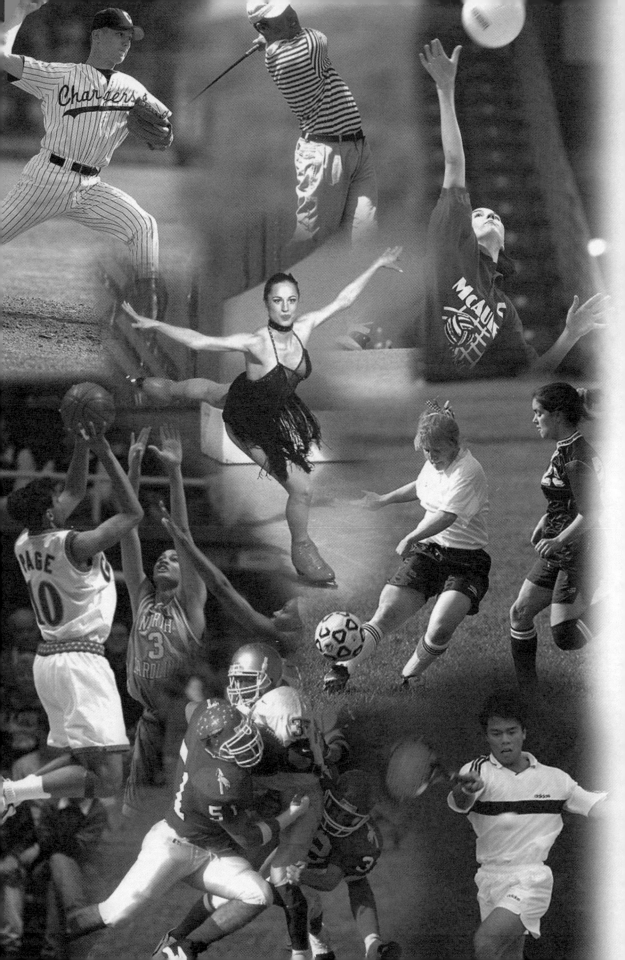

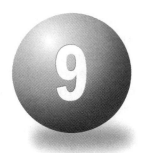

Functional Programs

The purpose of chapter 9 is to introduce you to some sample programs for specific sports, and the concepts that underly our thinking when we develop specific sport programs. As mentioned previously in the book, "the ball will provide you with a number of viable options to enhance your exercise toolkit." It is not meant to be the exclusive training apparatus for any kind of program. With this in mind, you will notice a number of free weight exercises that have not been described in *Strength Ball Training.* If you are unfamiliar with these exercises, we suggest you consult with a Certified Strength & Conditioning Specialist and or one of Human Kinetics other fine resources like the "Weight Training Steps To Success" series.

Football

Football, whether Canadian or American style, is an explosive sport. Throughout the game, players experience hard, purposeful hits. This places great stress on all joints.

The spine is sometimes placed in an awkward position as a result of these hits, which compounds stress to the joints. For these reasons the core must be prepared to absorb contacts. Training the body to adapt in a variety of planes and at different angles and speeds will result in stronger, more functional players. Power cleans will provide the stimulus for explosive power in the hips, while the medicine ball (MB) chest pass can develop the same type of power in the upper body. Protecting the shoulder is another key concern for the football player. The incline dumbbell (DB) press and prone row external rotation will develop the shoulders in the front and provide support from the back.

The following schedule is recommended for enhancing dynamic stability in preparation for playing football.

Football Day 1

Exercise	Sets	Repetitions
Power clean	4	5
Split squat	3	8
Romanian deadlift	4	6
Kneeling balance	4	60 seconds
Abdominal crunch	5	10

Football Day 2

Exercise	Sets	Repetitions
Push press	4	6
MB chest pass	5	8
Incline DB press	3	8
Bent over row	4	8
Prone row external rotation	3	8

Downhill Skiing

In downhill skiing, the top racers have been clocked at well over 60 miles per hour. Speeds of this nature make it difficult for the body to maintain its sport-specific position, especially while going in and out of turns. Downhill skiers must be able to hold the ski edges at these high speeds. It's important for the core and lower body to function as a linked system.

Another concern for a skier is the tremendous pressure placed on the hips and knees. The skier must have great strength and stability in these areas, especially to prevent injury. The back extension exercise will provide the static strength necessary for the lower back. In addition, the supine lower-abdominal curl and crunch will strengthen the abdomen, which must provide support for the core as well as transfer power throughout the body.

Downhill Skiing Day 1

Exercise	Sets	Repetitions
Snatch squat	4	6
Front squat	4	8
Back extension SB row	5	20
Leg curl	5	8
Supine lower-abdominal curl and crunch	4	10

Downhill Skiing Day 2

Exercise	Sets	Repetitions
Single-arm push press	3	6
DB bench press	3	10
Pull-up	3	Max. reps.
Scapular push-up	3	10
Sorinex Russian twist	4	12

Tennis

Tennis can be very hard on the body, as the dominant side always carries out the stroke. As a result of this, two types of injuries may occur: The dominant side may incur short, tight muscles as a result of the constant rotation to one side, and the non-dominant side may become weak from an unbalanced program. To counteract these possibilities, you will want to focus on twisting and turning movements for both sides of the body. The side-to-side rotation pass will allow the non-dominant side some training using explosive movements. In some cases, if your dominant side is significantly stronger than the opposite side, you may want to perform two to three extra sets for the weaker side.

From an upper-body perspective, the shoulder is one of the last links in the transfer of power from the legs and core to the racket. The DB presses and the isodynamic rear delt raise will develop the strength and stability in the shoulders for an explosive serve or return. Off-court conditioning can positively affect physical development and assist in injury prevention.

Tennis Day 1

Exercise	Sets	Repetitions
Lateral squat with ball push	3	12
Walking lunge and rotate	4	10
Kneeling balance, tennis-stroke move	5	60
Romanian deadlift	4	8
Standing calf raise	4	20
Side-to-side rotation pass	4	10

Tennis Day 2

Exercise	Sets	Repetitions
DB bench press	3	10
DB Arnold press	3	10
Lat pull-down, neutral grip	3	12
Isodynamic rear delt raise	3	10
Wrist curl and extension	3	12

Soccer

Successful soccer players require a combination of speed, explosion, and endurance. This combination requires development of the core and lower body, as reflected in the following program design. Too much emphasis on upper-body training will result in an increase in upper-body mass, which will raise the center of gravity. By emphasizing the lower body and increasing the muscle mass here, you can lower the center of gravity and increase the efficiency in running high-speed turns with the ball.

A soccer player must also be able to kick the ball with great power. Not only must the kicking leg be strong, but the planted leg must also be able to handle the stress and torque of the body on top of it. The lateral wall squat, with an inside leg-pivot position, is the most sport-specific exercise that a soccer player can perform. The MB soccer throw-in pass also provides an increase in power for both the legs and arms, which enhances throw-in ability. The following combination will provide a successful balance of the required elements.

Soccer Day 1

Exercise	Sets	Repetitions
Front squat	4	8
Lateral wall squat, inside leg	3	8
Reverse back extension	4	10
Single-leg curl	4	8
MB soccer throw-in pass	4	10
Calf raise	3	20

Soccer Day 2

Exercise	Sets	Repetitions
Push press	4	8
DB bench press	3	10
DB pull-over	3	12
Over-the-shoulder throw	3	8
MB supine Russian twist	3	12

Golf

Golf is very much like tennis in that overuse to the dominant side is an issue for many golfers. In the past, the most common training practice for golfers might have been to ride a stationary bike or jog a few miles in the off-season. These days, golfers take their game very seriously. The science of biomechanics has provided much-needed information for developing specific programs that address the muscle imbalances that are derived as a result of playing golf.

Balance and core strength will enhance the distance of your drives, while the upper-body exercises will provide the shoulder mobility necessary for swinging with greater ease. Restrictions in the shoulder and shoulder-blade movement during the swing can greatly affect accuracy. Another golf concern is posture, especially in the upper thoracic area. Exercises such as the hip extension knee flexion and the dumbbell step up will assist in restoring strength and mobility to the spine.

Golf Day 1

Exercise	Sets	Repetitions
Kneeling posterior shoulder stretch	4	60 seconds
DB step-up	3	10
Hip extension knee flexion	3	12
Leg curl	3	12
Cable axe chop	3	10
Russian twist	3	12

Golf Day 2

Exercise	Sets	Repetitions
Prone row external rotation	3	8
Seated rope row toward neck	3	10
DB pull-over	3	12
Back-to-back 180-degree rotation pass	3	10
Supine lower-abdominal cable curl	3	10

Judo

Judo is best known for both its spectacular throws and its grappling on the floor. These skills require speed and upper-body strength. By using the stability ball, you can emphasize the pulling muscles of the shoulder that are so important for those close confrontations. The supine pull-up is one exercise that will replicate the powerful co-contraction of all the posterior muscles and the core. It is possible to replicate an even more sport-specific movement by alternating the hand position or performing the exercises by holding onto a piece of cloth that is secured around a bar.

Many times during a round, one competitor will find himself out of balance and needing to fend off an attack. Great balance and strength are necessary for recovering and moving efficiently. The MB single-leg balance left-to-right exercise requires powerful movements combined with balance.

Judo Day 1

Exercise	Sets	Repetitions
Squat	4	8
Walking lunge and rotate	3	10
Romanian deadlift	3	6
Reverse back	3	12
MB single-leg balance, left to right	4	10
Jackknife	3	15

Judo Day 2

Exercise	Sets	Repetitions
Supine pull-up	3	10
MB push-up and pass	3	8
Bench press	3	10
Dip	3	Max. reps.
Standing biceps curl	3	10
Bridge T fall-off	3	12

Hockey

Ice hockey requires tremendous strength in the legs and core. Skillful execution and collision follow-through must utilize the upper-body musculature. In on-ice action, these muscle groups must work as an integrated unit to provide powerful movements.

Power cleans, supine pull-ups, and walk-outs into push-ups build the body together as a linked system. The squats and leg blasters develop the foundation of skating—great legs and hips.

Hockey uses high velocity, eccentric braking, and a rotational movement of the abdomen. Therefore, exercises that train the core in a standing position and through a transverse plane of movement (such as the side-to-side rotation pass and the back-to-back stop-and-go) predominate.

Shoulder-to-shoulder passes bring it all together, building upper-body power, core rotation strength, and linked system power, as the throw is initiated at the foot, transfers through the legs, moves into the hip and through the core, and follows through with the chest and arms.

Early in the off-season, complete these exercises with a low number of repetitions and controlled movements. Closer to the season, prescribe higher repetitions and explosive actions to improve speed and endurance. Hockey requires not just explosiveness but also repeated actions over the course of an entire game. In season, the program can be used twice a week for maintenance and for dynamic warm-ups.

Hockey Day 1

Exercise	Sets	Repetitions
Power clean	4	8
Split squat	3	20
Wall squat	3	12
Goldy's leg blaster	3	8
Back-to-back stop-and-go	3	20 each side
Standing ball-hug	3	20 taps
Side-to-side rotation pass	4	15

Hockey Day 2

Exercise	Sets	Repetitions
Walk-out into push-up	4	10
MB shoulder-to-shoulder pass	4	20
MB walk-over	3	8 each side
Supine pull-up	4	8
Prone row external rotation	3	8

Baseball

Baseball consists of quick bursts of action interspersed with rest. Success depends on the initiation of action and force delivery. Pitching, throwing, and batting mechanics draw upon standing core rotation, contralateral action, and weight transfer.

Running down balls, ball pick-ups, the run response from home plate, and base running all require great leg power, multi-directional movement capabilities, and a strong core. The baseball program features core rotation exercises, as well as complex exercises combining core rotation with lower- and upper-body strength requirements. Examples include the MB shoulder-to-shoulder pass and the walking lunge and rotate.

The single-arm push press, MB shoulder-to-shoulder pass, standing incline roll-out, and scapular push-up all link core strength while developing the posterior deltoid and rotator cuff muscle groups. Leg variations provide standard squat power, lateral squat movement, and stride power through walking lunges.

Baseball players need to use a low number of repetitions to build strength and hypertrophy. Exercises should be completed through a full range of motion to develop dynamic flexibility. Closer to the season, explosive power predominates. The abdominals should be set for all exercises. Exercises requiring full-body multi-joint action and rotation should feature a powerful initiation of force from the core and hip region.

Baseball Day 1

Exercise	Sets	Repetitions
Lateral squat with ball push	4	6 each leg
Front squat	4	8
Walking lunge and rotate	4	15 each leg
Bridge with MB drop	3	10 each side
Back-to-back stop-and-go	3	10 each side
Russian twist	4	10

Baseball Day 2

Exercise	Sets	Repetitions
Single-arm push press	3	6
MB shoulder-to-shoulder pass	3	10
Standing two-ball roll-out	2	Max. reps.
Supine pull-up	3	Max. reps.
Scapular push-up	3	10
Sorinex Russian twist	4	12

Figure Skating

Figure skating is either done individually or in pairs. Both require the skater to perform a short program (2 minutes 40 seconds) and a long program (approximately 3 to 4 minutes) during a competition. During each program, specific elements must be performed, requiring difficult footwork, spins, and jumps. The metabolic demands are intense, and skaters must be capable of precise biomechanical performance even toward the end of a program.

The standing progression of the kneeling side pass, the MB single-leg balance, left-to-right exercise, and the walking lunge and rotate help prepare for the torso rotation necessary in entering and leaving jumps, spins, and complex footwork sequences. A strong core is required for landing and stopping as well, so bridge T fall-offs and standing two-ball roll-outs are included to accelerate the demands on the core.

Skaters' legs must be strong and able to generate power far into a program. Skaters should develop their musculature with a moderate number of repetitions (8 to 10). This is later built into high-repetition leg prescription, increasing to 20, then 30, then 40, and finally 50 repetitions to a set in the final stage of preparation. This phase is followed by a tapering cycle in which skaters maintain their strength and endurance, yet have adequate recovery and regeneration time to enter competitions fit and rested. The leg blaster, walking lunges, and split squat combine to strengthen the hips and legs.

Figure skaters spend a great deal of time on one leg and also must land properly, so balance and single-leg exercises were selected. The MB single-leg balance left-to-right exercise, kneeling on the ball, and split squats are helpful in this regard.

Figure Skating Day 1

Exercise	Sets	Repetitions
Squat	4	6
Walking lunge and rotate	3	10
Goldy's leg blaster	3	8
Split squat	3	8
Reverse back extension	3	12
MB single-leg balance, left to right	4	10
Jackknife	3	15
Kneel on ball	3	60 seconds
Bridge T fall-off	2	12 each side

Figure Skating Day 2

Exercise	Sets	Repetitions
Supine pull-up	3	10
Incline pull-down	3	8
Cable fly	2	10
Standing two-ball roll-out	3	10
MB push-up and pass	2	10
Kneeling side pass, standing progression	3	10

Cross-Country Skiing

In cross-country skiing, the aerobic system is worked at peak performance, always toying with tapping into the anaerobic lactate system. The anaerobic threshold is reached when a skier passes, skis up an incline, and sprints to the finish line. A strong core is critical for success. An athlete's ability to ski over challenging terrain relies on the power of the core. The core is also the speed center, and it determines the efficiency of upper-body action.

A cross-country skier must propel herself over the snow. This requires a kick phase, which also utilizes the arms contralaterally for forward propulsion. Split squats, leg blasters, and leg curls have been selected for leg strength, beginning with a moderate number of repetitions (10 to 15). The final preparation phase builds leg endurance with exercises such as the split squat prescription of two-minute sets with maximum repetitions. Note that athletes must progressively build up to a two-minute set in order to minimize Delayed Onset of Muscle Soreness (DOMS).

The standing two-ball roll-out, dumbbell pull-over, supine pull-up, and cable fly exercises combine to develop the link between the chest and back, and arm action and core stability. Other exercises further serve to build muscles around the core for injury-prevention and performance purposes.

Cross-Country Skiing Day 1

Exercise	Sets	Repetitions
Split squat	4	2 minutes
Goldy's leg blaster	3	15
Leg curl	3	12
Jackknife	3	12
Reverse back extension	3	10
Russian twist	3	12

Cross-Country Skiing Day 2

Exercise	Sets	Repetitions
Standing two-ball roll-out	3	12
Triceps blaster	2	10
DB pull-over	3	12
Supine pull-up	3	10
Cable fly	3	10

Basketball

Basketball is a read-and-react game of stops and starts, vertical jumps, and agility. Multi-directional movement is needed to be creative on offense and effective on defense. Of course, lateral movement is a common necessity for all positions.

Forwards and low posts have to be powerful to box out, set screens, and rebound. Guards must work hard to set up plays and hustle back on defense. They must be able to run backward quickly as well as demonstrate high-speed agility.

Squat jumps, lateral squats, walking lunges, and split squats combine to prepare the player to run, jump, and move laterally. The full-body multi-joint MB pass integrates leg and hip power with a powerful chest pass.

The side-to-side rotation passes, shoulder-to-shoulder passes, and over-the-shoulder throws build the abdominal muscles in a transverse plane of movement while linking in the arm action needed for effective passing.

Upper-body exercises such as walk-arounds, medicine ball walk-overs, and MB chest passes increase chest and back strength while developing the posterior shoulder and rotator cuff muscle groups to prevent injury. These exercises require independent arm action and a strong core.

Building a linked system helps with skill execution, while upper-body and core strength help players battle in contact situations.

Basketball Day 1

Exercise	Sets	Repetitions
Lateral squat with ball push	3	8
Walking lunge and rotate	4	12
Split squat	3	15
Full-body multi-joint MB pass	5	8
Standing calf raise	4	20
Side-to-side rotation pass	3	10
Over-the-shoulder throw	3	10

Basketball Day 2

Exercise	Sets	Repetitions
DB bench press	3	10
Ball walk-around	4	360 degrees
MB walk-over	3	8 each side
MB shoulder-to-shoulder pass	3	10
Incline pull-down	3	12
MB chest pass	5	6

Volleyball

Volleyball players must be able to react quickly and move explosively off the ground to spike, block, and dive. Players must be able to attain height during jumps while still effectively covering ground to position themselves for plays. Players stay low while engaged in this position, using forward, backward, and lateral shuffles. Lower-body power, single-leg balance, and shoulder strength are essential.

The volleyball program builds leg power and vertical explosiveness through single-leg box jump-ups, front squats, lateral wall squats, and full-body multi-joint passes. These exercises develop leg and hip strength plus the countermovement needed for quickness and vertical jumps.

Superior core strength is developed with descending bench roll-outs (a great exercise for tall athletes with long torsos), over-the-shoulder throws, and the MB single-leg balance, left-to-right exercise. The upper-body exercises link many muscle groups together and serve to activate the core muscles as well as build strength without hypertrophy.

Volleyball players begin with a low to moderate number of repetitions (6 to 12) to build strength and a solid foundation. These repetitions are then increased (such as the full-body multi-joint MB pass prescription of 20 repetitions per set) to build strength endurance and combine strength training with energy-system training. Closer to the competitive season, the number of repetitions is reduced to two or three for pure power, and between-set rest intervals are reduced as well.

Volleyball Day 1

Exercise	Sets	Repetitions
Single-leg box jump-ups	3	6
Front squat	4	8
Lateral wall squat	3	8
Full-body multi-joint MB pass	3	20
Over-the-shoulder throw	3	10
Bench roll-outs	4	12
MB single-leg balance, left-to-right	3	10
Calf raise	4	20

Volleyball Day 2

Exercise	Sets	Repetitions
Push press	5	8
DB pull-over	5	12
Shoulder-to-shoulder pass	5	12
Russian twist	3	12
MB push-up and pass	3	10

Bibliography

Berg, K. 1989. Balance and its measure in the elderly: A review. *Physiotherapy* 41:240-246.

Cholewicki, J. et al. 1996. Mechanical stability of the in vivo lumbar spine: Implications for injury and chronic low back pain. *Clinical Biomechanics* 11(1).

Chu, D. 1992. *Jumping into plyometrics*. Champaign, IL: Leisure Press.

Irrgang, J. et al. 1994. Balance and proprioception training for rehabilitation of the lower extremity. *Journal of Sport Rehabilitation* 3.

Lephart, S. et al. 1997. The role of proprioception in the management and rehabilitation of athletic injuries. *American Journal of Sports Medicine* 25(1).

———. 1998. Anatomy and physiology of proprioception and neuromuscular control. *Athletic Therapy Today* 3(5).

McGill. 1998. Low back exercises: Evidence for improving exercise regimes. *Physical Therapy* 78(7).

Posner-Mayer, J. 1995. *Swiss ball applications for orthopedic and sports medicine*. Denver: Ball Dynamics International.

Richardson, C. et al. 1999. *Therapeutic exercise for spinal segmental stabilization in low back pain*. Edinburgh: Churchill Livingtone.

Twist, P. 2001. *Complete conditioning for ice hockey*. Champaign, IL: Human Kinetics.

Wirhed, R. 1990. *Athletic ability and the anatomy of motion*. London: Wolfe Medical Publications.

For More Information

Questions for the Authors

If you have furthur questions for the authors or are interested in beginning your own strength ball training program, please contact the authors at the addresses listed below.

Lorne Goldenberg
Strength Tek Fitness & Wellness Consultants at www.strengthtek.com
The Athletic Conditioning Center at www.accottawa.com.
613-820-9682
Strength Tek Fitness & Wellness Consultants
1010 Morrison Dr.
Ottawa, Ont, Canada K2H 8K7

Peter Twist
Twist Conditioning Incorporated www.sport-specific.com
info@sport-specific.com
604-904-6556
Twist Conditioning Incorporated
1803 Welch Street
North Vancouver, British Columbia, Canada V7P 1B7

Products
To purchase ABS stability balls and medicine balls, visit Twist Conditioning Inc. online store through www.sport-specific.com or email products@sport-specific.com to receive a catalogue. You may also call directly toll free 888-214-4244 (outside North America call 604-904-6556).

Ball Seminars and Consultation
Contact Lorne Goldenberg at 613-820-9682 or Peter Twist at 604-904-6556 or info@sport-specific.com.

Conditioning Camps
Contact Lorne Goldenberg's Athlete Conditioning Center at 613-820-9682 or www.strengthtek.com. Contact Peter Twist's Conditioning and Athlete Development Camps at 604-904-6556 or camps@sport-specific.com.

About the Authors

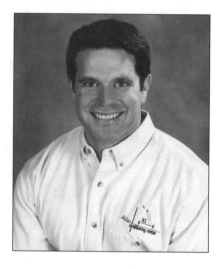

Lorne Goldenberg has worked with professional athletes as a strength and conditioning coach with four National Hockey League (NHL) teams, Team Canada's hockey team, and football players in the Canadian Football League (CFL). He lectures internationally on stability ball exercises and program integration for such groups as the National Strength and Conditioning Association, Society of Weight Training Injury Specialists, provincial associations, and professional teams. He has written for the NSCA *Journal of Strength and Conditioning, Ironman, Physical, Men's Journal,* and the *Journal of Hockey Conditioning and Player Development,* which he also owns.

Goldenberg is the president and director of conditioning at Strength Tek Fitness & Wellness Consultants, a group of more than 100 employees in four Canadian cities, and at the Athletic Conditioning Center. He lives in Ottawa, Ontario, with his wife, Julie, and their children, Isaak and Danielle. In his free time he enjoys traveling to the beach with family and collecting Batman comic books and paraphernalia.

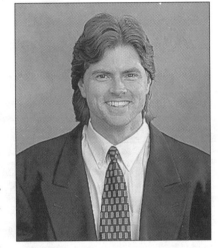

Peter Twist has coached in the NHL for nine years and is currently the strength and conditioning coach for the Vancouver Canucks as well as President of the Hockey Conditioning Coaches Association. An exercise physiologist and sport scientist, he is co-editor of the *Journal of Hockey Conditioning and Player Development*, author of *Complete Hockey Conditioning*, co-author of *The Physiology of Ice Hockey*, and an author in *High-Performance Sports Conditioning*.

Twist has published over 100 papers and is a frequent guest lecturer at international conferences, seminars, coaching clinics and university courses on topics such as coaching, quickness and agility, core power, and sport conditioning. His revolutionary training concepts have been well received by thousands of coaches and trainers throughout the world. In recognition of his contribution to the field of strength and conditioning, Twist was the 1998 recipient of the National Strength and Conditioning Association's President's Award.

Twist is also the owner of Twist Conditioning Incorporated (see **www.sport-specific.com**) and Peter Twist's Conditioning and Athlete Development Camps. Twist has coached over 700 professional athletes, including Hakeem Olajuwon of the Toronto Raptors, Pavel Bure of the Florida Panthers, and Mark Messier of the New York Rangers. Each summer over 500 elite athletes from high school, college, and professional ranks attend his camps.

Twist is an NSCA-certified strength and conditioning specialist and a former NSCA provincial director for British Columbia. He lives in Vancouver, Canada in the north shore mountains with his wife Julie. Together with their daughters, Zoe and Mackenzie, and dogs, Rico and Loosy, they enjoy mountain hiking, descent running, snowshoeing, black diamond tree skiing, and, of course, hot tubbing.

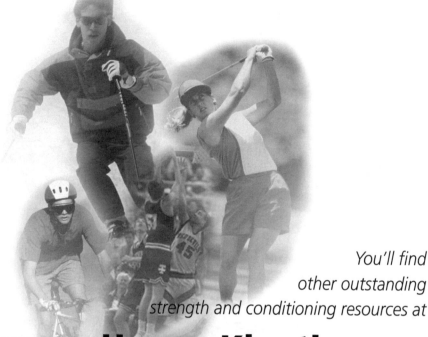

You'll find
other outstanding
strength and conditioning resources at

www.HumanKinetics.com

In the U.S. call

800-747-4457

Australia	08 8277 1555
Canada	800-465-7301
Europe	+44 (0) 113 255 5665
New Zealand	09-523-3462

 HUMAN KINETICS
The Premier Publisher for Sports and Fitness
P.O. Box 5076 • Champaign, IL 61825-5076 USA